Hospice Care At Home

by Starr Calo-oy with Bob Calo-oy

Foreword by Mitchell F. Finnie M.D.

A Guide to Caring for Your Dying Loved One at Home

Readers Praise

"If you are in need of a resource to help guide you with home hospice care for your loved one, look no further. Starr details many important topics for providing compassionate and competent bedside care, managing the "good death", and dealing with loss. Congratulations Starr, your experience shines throughout and it will help those in need!"

Dr. Dennis S. Pacl
Extra Care Palliative Consultants

"Starr has written a remarkable account of her practical hands-on experience coupled with great love and compassion and this proves to be a winning combination. She takes the experience a step further by showing the reader how to easily do the same."

Bernadine Dailey
Odyssey Healthcare
Hospice Administrator

"Starr & Bob cared for my wife for a year and a half before she passed away in their home. I have witnessed, first hand, their tender loving patience and highly knowledgeable methods in daily practice. I have especially appreciated that Starr has accurately related what to expect in my wife's decline and how to handle it emotionally. She has poured the knowledge gained from her many years of intimate contact with terminally ill patients and their hurting families into this book and I highly recommend it to anyone needing to understand more about home hospice care."

Dr. Charles A. Belfi, M.A., Ph.D.

"This guide should be a mandatory item in every Hospice Kit given to caregivers by the admitting hospice nurse. As a Hospice Chaplain, I have seen caregivers and entire families struggle, in ignorance, over the dying process and the care of their loved one. The gentle and practical suggestions offered to prepare for the death event as well what to expect in the days that follow will be truly appreciated. This guide will be a blessing to the patient, the caregiver and the entire hospice family!"

Deacon Ernest Roy Amo MA

Christus Santa Rosa Hospice

Hospice Care at Home

Hospice Care
At Home

by Starr Calo-oy with Bob Calo-oy

Published by Orchard Publications

P.O. Box 680815

San Antonio, Texas 78268

www.caregiversadvice.net

First Edition 2006

ISBN # 0-9753195-1-5

Printed in the United States of America

Hospice (2) Hospice Home Care (3) Dying at Home (4) Funeral Planning (5) Aging Parents (6) Dying (7) Death (8) Alzheimer's Disease (9) Consultations (10) Care Tips (11) Choking

Table of Contents

Dedication

This book is first and foremost dedicated to our Heavenly Father who always holds us in the palm of His hand while we are on Earth and then gently calls us home to live with Him.

And, in loving memory of our mother,
Virginia Sue Turner,
who came to our home for hospice care in August 2006 and blessed all of us with her great faith and love for Jesus.

"For me to live is Christ, and to die is gain."
Philippians 1:21

Acknowledgements

We want to thank you Linda Johnson-Sailer, our best friend, for patiently teaching us hospice care with our very first patient 17 years ago. If it weren't for you, we would not have written our books. We love you!

I thank our mother, Virginia Turner, who is surely in heaven now, for editing our manuscript again. I am so grateful to her for allowing us to care for her the last few weeks of her life. Thank you daddy (Bob Turner) for being a devoted, loving and caring husband to our mother for 52 years, believing in what we do and always encouraging us to do more.

Charles (Dr. Charles A. Belfi), you have been a remarkable blessing to our family ever since you first brought your wife, Eufrasia, into our care. Thank you for sponsoring our writing, editing our book and for accepting us as your family. We love you so much!

God bless hospice agencies everywhere for all of their tender loving care, compassionate patience with hurting families, rich experience and much needed wisdom and their willingness to share it. We especially want to thank Vista Care Hospice, Christus Santa Rosa

Hospice and Vitas Hospice for all of their guidance and help over the years.

Mark Mayfield (of Litho Press): You are a dear friend, a great photographer and have a keen eye for detail! Thank you for the gift of photographing our book cover and helping with the final details. You also had incredible patience with us while we worked on the production of our book. Thank you once again for helping us, once again, to produce our work so beautifully.

Our two children still at home, Khalea, age 9 and Khaiyan, age 11, were so very patient while I worked late hours and weekends writing and I thank them with all of my heart for sharing their mommy!

Thank you Dr. Finnie for writing our foreword, treating our hospice patients at home and being our advisor for so long. You are a blessing.

Jackie Johnson (Marketing Director at Kingsley Place, Medical Center), thank you for being such a good friend and hosting our CAPS (Children of Aging Parents Support Group).

Foreword
by
Mitchell F. Finnie MD.

Before the 1960's, families cared for their own dying loved ones at home in lieu of hospitalization. Nursing homes did not exist. It became necessary for there to be a qualified place for the ailing elderly when men went off to war and wives had to take over their husbands' jobs, therefore nursing homes became the alternative to hospitalization. As time went by, modern working families completely moved away from caring for their elderly and dying loved ones

When I first began my medical training, hospice care was just starting to be recognized as a beneficial tool. In days prior, it was not uncommon for patients with terminal illnesses to be shuttled down a hospital corridor to a remote room to be left alone to die. Often, the diagnosis was not discussed with the patient and hospital personnel minimized contact with the terminally ill. Unfortunately, as a result many people died a lonely death. Most family members had never been exposed to death, much less experienced the process of someone dying in their home.

The word hospice comes from the Latin word "hospis", meaning host and guest. Hospice is the root word for hospitality, hospital, hotel, hostel and hospice in English. A large part of hospice care was bringing the American family back to the dying process.

Fortunately, hospice care has become increasingly common over the past two decades. The pendulum has swung back to patients staying at home during their dying days. An entire generation did not experience family members dying at home.

Working with various hospice agencies, I have seen hundreds of hospice patients. The vast majority spend their final days in their own home, or in the home of a loved one. As a physician, I tend to see the patients and families when there are difficulties for the patient to remain home during the death process. At times, loved ones can be reassured by caring for them at home, that the proper care is being provided. Other times, a hospital setting is required to put the family members at ease or to control symptoms of the patient.

From my experience, educating family members about the dying process is critical. *"Hospice Care at Home"* is an invaluable tool for families to assist in the care of their loved ones who spend their final days at home. The practical nature of the book serves as a wonderful resource for family members and loved ones.

Starr and Bob, who specialize in hospice care in their own home, have accumulated a wealth of hands-on experience over the past 17 years, which is evident in the practical details of the book. Because this information shared is from personal experience, it is genuine and down-to-earth, and will educate and enlighten the reader on the true meaning of hospice.

The concrete details of the book gently and effectively walk the family caregiver through the death process. Such practical information as the physical signs of dying, working with funeral homes, what to do on the day of the loved one's death and steps to take after the funeral, are related from personal experience and serve to educate the reader caring for a loved one in a home setting. Anyone who provides care for a loved one who is dying at home should possess a copy of their book.

Not only do family members need such practical information, but also those in the health profession. The knowledge to be gained from the book will benefit doctors, nurses, chaplains, social workers and other members of the hospice health care team. Any physician who provides primary care has a need for the information provided in *"Hospice Care at Home"* in order to gain personal insight of one-on-one caregiving, 24/7.

It has required tremendous strides for our society to return the dying process to the homefront. People are desperate for resources to help them provide care for their loved ones in their final days because they simply don't know how. Starr's book provides this information. It helps one understand the role hospice plays and the unique roles of each member of the hospice team.

Fortunately, death is once again being treated as part of the life cycle and is being brought back into the home. It can be a frightening and intimidating task, but with the help of the hospice agency and books such as this, people are staying home in their final days and experiencing reassuring comfort in being with those who love them most. The greatest gift someone can give is allowing a loved one to die in a family, friendly, home environment.

If you will take the suggestions and practical advice provided in this book to heart and apply them, you can more easily give this gift to your loved one.

When all has been said and done, as you look back on this season in your life, you will experience great satisfaction in knowing that you were there when it meant the most.

Introduction

(Note: *The suggestions in this book are based on the assumption that all are agreed that your loved one, hereafter referred to as "LO", will die at home in your care. Also, the authors have chosen to use the pronoun "him" instead of "him/her". All book content refers to both men & women*)

When Bob and I first started caring for the elderly in our home seventeen years ago, my mother asked me if I was sure I wanted to care for people who were going to die in our home. Being a concerned mother, she thought the work might depress me.

My answer to her was that God had called us to do this particular type of caregiving and where He sends you, He gives you the grace to carry it out and joyfully so! This remains true all of these years later. We truly enjoy every facet of our work and ministry to the patients we care for and their families.

There is nothing compared to being privileged enough to share the last few days of a person's life. We derive such satisfaction from knowing that we have made a difference in their family's lives also. When we wake up each day, we look forward to what the new day holds for us and when we close our eyes at night, after a long days' work, we have a Godly pride in what we accomplished and the lives we touched that day.

Since the tragedy occurred when the trade centers were destroyed in 2001, Americans have been returning to patriotism, home and hearth in most every area of their lives. We are pleased to see that a growing respect for our elderly is one of these areas.

For five decades, we as a country gradually moved away from caring for our own dying at home. We have been inundated with modern technology and just haven't even considered much of anything else but to make money and accumulate things. Relationships with our youth, elderly, sickly and in many cases even our own marriages have been last on our list of priorities. The result? The highest divorce rate, teenage suicide and pregnancies and runaways in history.

The very foundation of our country was built on biblical principals, one of them being that if you honor your mother and father, things will go well for you and you shall live long upon the earth. The elderly are living longer because of the new technology and they honored and revered the wisdom of their parents. The youth are dying younger because they don't. But the good news is that we are waking up and repenting.

Every time you turn on the news you hear about another group which has been formed to reinstate the morals our great country was built on. Old Glory is flying high once again and we are taking our country back.

Most people just don't know how to care for their dying loved ones at home or where to look for help. Because you need a degree for most any job these days, most families are under the mistaken idea that in order for them to do hospice care at home, they need to be qualified. The idea doesn't even enter their mind because subconsciously they fear they might make a fatal mistake and that terminal care should be performed by doctors, nurses and hospitals.

Don't get me wrong. We appreciate the medical professionals who specialize in the dying process and their help is needed. I'm only saying that there is more than one way to help your terminally ill LO.

The purpose of our book is to teach families who want to be with their loved ones at home for their last days on earth, as opposed to a more institutional setting, how to provide that care and how to do it exceptionally.

We can't blow the proverbial horn loud enough for the many hospice agencies that have stepped up to the plate over the past fifty years. They excel in compassion, knowledge, patience and work hand-in-hand with the family to provide a pain and symptom free climate at home for the dying.

As we get up in age and our needs change, out of necessity, our residences must change too. The trend for the elderly, until recently, has been:

1. From living at home
2. To a small apartment
3. To an independent retirement community
4. To an independent living facility
5. To an assisted living facility
6. To a family member's home
7. To a nursing home or
8. A personal care home
9. To the hospital
10. To the cemetery

Our goal in writing this book is to show the family how to take care of their own relatives at home when they decide that this is the route they want to take. If we can eliminate the fear of inadequacy that comes with terminal care, then we have met our goal.

We aren't saying this will be easy and that it's for everyone but if you want to learn how to care for your LO throughout the dying process, you are holding the right book in your hands to do just that.

Welcome to the rewarding world of terminal homecare!

Chapter One

The Diagnosis – What Now?

As adult children, we have always believed that we would probably outlive our parents, so when we find out that one of our parents is dying, we automatically accept it, right?

Or is this the case? You have been married to your spouse for 50 something years. Even though you have always said that you will both go together (both of you will just lie down one day, close your eyes and pass away quietly-together), when the doctor says he/she will be going on ahead of you, you just quietly accept it, right again?

No! We cannot wrap our mind around the inconceivable thought that we are soon going to be left behind! After all, that wasn't the plan. We still had so many things to do with our LO. It's just not fair. Wait a minute. Surely there is something we can do about this.

We have usually been able to change things to turn out the way we want them. As human beings, we are natural-born problem solvers. When we haven't personally experienced the finality of death and someone we love dearly is faced with this irreversible situation, we shrink from it and, yes, deny its very existence.

If we feel this way, imagine what our LO must be going through (if they are well-minded)! The sad part of it all is that usually your LO doesn't want to upset you or other family members so they don't talk about their feelings. They just keep all their fears and grief bottled up inside and become withdrawn and depressed.

Usually, people first get the "bad news" at the doctor's office or in the hospital so they aren't alone to adequately evaluate and absorb the initial shock until later. The doctor will have given your LO his own suggestions as to care options for the future, however it will be up to him and the family how the future will actually be handled.

You may or may not have been with him when he received the news. If you were, he would probably still be talking about it when you both left the doctor's presence.

Timing is very important in every area of our lives and even more so now. You don't want to say anything that would cause him to clam up but you do want him to know that you will be here for him for the long haul without making him feel guilty about burdening you.

Our suggestion is to simply let him talk if he wants to. If he chooses to be silent, respect that as well.

Please remember this: there is no right or wrong way of handling this awkward situation if you handle it with love. However there are a few don'ts:

1. **Don't** try and force your LO to cheer up or prevent him from crying.
2. **Don't** force your LO to talk about dying if he doesn't want to.
3. **Don't** allow him to overhear you whispering about him to someone else. In doing so, you would invalidate his sanity, authority and very presence.
4. **Don't** start avoiding him because of your own pain or tears. He needs you now more than ever.
5. **Don't** cry harder and longer than he does in his presence. This is about him, not you.
6. **Don't** start making plans without his input unless he has dementia.

Express your love for him and ask his forgiveness if there is anything between the two of you. After the first tears have been shed, discuss pain management, hospice alternatives, funeral arrangements, any family, friends and clergy he wants to come see him and when.

Don't be taken off guard if he starts talking about who he wants to will his personal effects to and his plans. Remember, he has just lost control of his life. Making plans may be his way of feeling in control of something, even if it is only materially. Get out a pen and paper and offer to take notes for him. Go with the flow. Don't try to stop him.

He may ask you to tell the other family members for him. He may express a concern about his finances. So many things must go through someone's mind when they find out that their time is short and they can think of a jillion things they still have to accomplish before they leave. The main thing at this point is for you to reassure him that you will help him with everything he wants to do and not to worry. He can depend on you.

When your LO has dementia

If your LO isn't aware that he is going to die, there is no good thing that can come from your informing him. He probably will not understand. If you are crying when you tell him, it can cause him to get depressed, frightened or combative. He won't even know why anyway.

Instead, share your feelings with other family members and close friends after you make plans yourself and enlist their help while you're at it.

Love on him, make him comfortable and tell him all the positive things you have been holding back. Now is the time.

Surround yourself with the memories that bonded you together and then share them with others who care.

You may need to busy yourself, as his primary caregiver, with last minute details, if there is time.

Make your time count. Plan this so that you will be proud of yourself when it's all over. No regrets.

There will be different things you will want to do with and for him, depending on which stage of dementia he is in at the time he is diagnosed, and his capability for activity.

If he is in early stage and still able to comprehend what lies ahead, he may want to document his feelings and messages to his loved ones on video before he enters the next stage. This can be quite therapeutic for all of you.

However, if he is in the latter stages, you will be so occupied with his care that you really won't have much time to do anything but care for him.

Regardless of the situation, be sure to surround yourself with family and friends that have a caring, compassionate heart and want to help with what you and your LO are facing.

You are going to need the support.

Chapter Two
Interview with Your Loved One

If your LO is able to hold an intelligent conversation with you and has no communication problems, ask him about the following: (it would be wise to tape him audibly or better yet, to video tape this conversation)

If the LO is your parent, you've got to get past feeling like a child and intruding on his privacy. Now is the time for action, and neither one of you have a choice. These things must be done. It's extremely important that you work on all of this before you get too busy caregiving and your LO is completely incapacitated to help you take care of business. The following is a list of questions to go over with him:

1) Who is your family attorney? Where can I find his contact information?

2) Do you have a power of attorney? Who is it? I need his contact information. (If not, ask him to appoint you. If he agrees, make sure his attorney understands the type of POA you need to carry out his wishes and to have access to all of his holdings for his future care. The POA expires at the time of his death)

You need to have the POA notarized in the presence of two witnesses who do not have any interest in his affairs. The attorney will go into more detail regarding the rules. If he already has a POA and wants to keep this person as his POA, get with him to make sure he has all of the following information. If your LO wants to appoint a different POA, for example yourself, get with his attorney and tell him so. Then ask your LO the following questions:

1. Do you have a financial planner or an accountant? Where can I find his contact information?

2. Tell me where all of your bank accounts are. I need all of the passwords, balances and account numbers.

3. Do you have a current will; where is it and is it exactly the way you want it? (If he says he wants to update it, call his attorney and make an appointment for your LO to talk to him)

4. Where is your marriage certificate? (ask this if your LO's spouse is still living. You will need this so you can help him/her file for benefits after your LO dies)

5. What current life insurance do you have? Where are the policies? Have you been dealing with a particular agent? Where is the contact information located?

6. Do you have funeral insurance? Where do you keep the paperwork?

7. Do you have funeral arrangements made with a specific funeral home? Where is all of your paperwork located?

8. I need a list of all of your current credit cards and the passwords and balances on each.

9. Do you own any property I don't know about? I need the details.

10. Do you have a safe deposit box? I need to know where it's located, the password and account number.

11. Do you have a pension or retirement plan with any of your former employers? Who are they and how do I contact them?

12. Do you have any CD's or IRA's? Who do you have them with?

13. I need you to help me list all of your assets and debts.

Place all of this information in a separate folder for future reference. This will take time to gather but you must have the information at your fingertips at any given time so get it done. Don't put it off. Depending on your LO's level of strength, it may take quite a few interviews, so start early.

If your LO has dementia or cannot communicate with you for this information, you need to initiate a search of his home and/or office. Enlist the help and legwork of your family. You may need to divide up the list among several people. Call a family meeting with a few of the more organized and diligent members. Schedule the next meeting with them (have them bring their weekly planners or calendars with them) before they leave. Tell them that you will all report on your findings at the next meeting.

This may sound like a lot of unnecessary work but if you've never been through it, you have no idea how important it is to get it done right. If you have been through it and not been this organized, then you will appreciate our attention to the small details.

Chapter Three
Planning the Funeral

It would seem that once the caregiving is over, it's all downhill, but that isn't the case.

Now comes an avalanche of paperwork, planning and imminent decisions to be made. Accept offers to help as they come. If you don't have a plan, you will miss out on that help because you won't know what there is to help with.

That's what this chapter is all about and that's why it's in the beginning of our book; so that you don't overlook the plans that need to be made far in advance. The care will be addressed later on in the book. At this point, the authors assume the position that your LO is still living and you are looking for information on how to handle the entire dying process; both emotionally and factually, so let's get started.

What to do Immediately After Diagnosis

Select the funeral home:

Your family may have always used a particular funeral home or perhaps you have never had any experience dealing with one. If your LO already has arrangements made, ask him where the paperwork is and review it to see what is included and if there is any balance owed. If your LO has dementia and cannot communicate with him, search his home for any important paperwork such as funeral arrangements, insurance policies and bank information. You may feel as if you are violating his privacy but it's time to step up to the plate and take over. This is a great service you are performing for your family and LO. If there is no funeral home preference, you can ask friends or family for a referral and call to make an appointment.

Make an appointment to see the funeral director:

Once you have located the paperwork, call the funeral home and find out if all arrangements are in order. If so, make an appointment with a funeral director to plan the funeral.

The obituary:

If you want to save money, write the obituary and arrange to have it placed in the newspaper yourself. The funeral home will gladly do it for you, but it will cost more. Call the newspaper and ask for the obituaries department. Ask them how much they charge by the word and for a picture. You will be surprised how expensive this is. Get your family to pitch in for the cost if your LO does not have any money. If he does have money, have him pay for it. Talk to him about it, if he is lucid and stable enough and ask him what he would want in his obituary. This may sound strange to you at first, but it can be very therapeutic for both of you. Planning the funeral gives your LO a certain element of control over his seemingly uncontrollable life while at the same time reassuring you both that things will go exactly the way he wants them to go.

Write the obituary or have the writer in your family write it and then make several copies and place them in a manila folder for later. Once this is out of the way, you'll have one less thing to do.

List of friends & family to notify:

Start making a list of people to call about the date planned for the viewing and funeral. Go through your LO's address book and, if possible, talk it over with him. There may be certain individuals he doesn't want you to include. Don't make him explain. Just accept his decision. Write down their names, addresses (including zips for later when you send thank you cards for the flowers etc.) and phone numbers. Make 3 copies and place them in a folder.

Eulogy:

Talk with your family and decide who will be delivering the eulogy. This person needs to begin gathering the facts about your LO now and compose the speech. Stay on top of this, asking them from time to time if it has been completed. Ask for a copy, make several of your own and file them in their own folder. It's never too early to get this ready.

Select the music:

Talk to your family and ask them if they would like a particular soloist, organist or tape to be played for the funeral. Decide between you if you want lyric sheets to be provided.

If your LO is still relatively lucid, you might want to ask him about his song choices. If this is a parent, he might have a favorite song about children or about the joys of being a parent or it may even be a love song both of your parents enjoyed throughout their lives. If he isn't lucid enough to talk to about this, a family member may have unique knowledge about his preferences.

Officiating;

Your LO may have his own pastor or priest who has looked out for his spiritual welfare for a while. If your LO has a preference for the person to officiate his funeral, then ask him/her. You will need to supply this person with a copy of the agenda and a fact sheet on your LO. After the funeral, it is customary to give this person an honorarium of $50.00 to $100.00 depending on the extent of his involvement.

If he has not been active for many years but would like someone who knows the Lord to officiate but doesn't know anyone, you or another family member need to suggest your own pastor or priest.

If your LO does not believe in God at all, you might consider one of your more outspoken family members to write the eulogy and perform a memorial service at the funeral home chapel and then have a graveside service. Then again, the attendees could be directed that the service is over when you are finished in the chapel and then let the funeral home carry out the burial from there.

Location

Where to hold the service needs to be decided; church, funeral chapel or home. If he has been active in church and has a relationship with the pastor or priest, talk to him about officiating. It's important that your LO be consulted if he can still relate his wishes. That's why we strongly suggest that you commit these plans to writing at the time of diagnosis, before things get complicated. Certainly, it's very difficult to plan a funeral for someone you dearly love while he is alive, but consider the alternative; it's much harder right after they pass away.

Are you going to have a viewing the night before? If so, where? The decision about the location may depend on this answer. The funeral home usually can provide this and if your LO has arrangements already made with them, it may be included with what he has already paid but don't assume anything- ask.

If there is not going to be any service at all or your LO wants cremation without any kind of ceremony, consider a family/friend gathering at home and start by reminiscing about his life (see Chapter Ten for alternatives). You could have video footage going on in the background for the duration of the event. Keep it light, humorous and honoring. This is not the time to share any negative happenings during his life.

Method

Has your LO requested to be cremated or buried? If cremation is his choice, does he want a viewing beforehand? If so, he will need to be embalmed first. How about a memorial service in lieu of a regular funeral service? How does he want his remains handled?

If he is to be buried, does he want a graveside service?

Pallbearers

The pallbearers need to be selected, asked and written down with full contact information. Plan on 6-8 people.

Date and day

Are there out-of-town guests or family to wait for? If so, remember that the funeral does not have to take place immediately. Talk to your funeral director for the specifics. Make the calls to those who want to attend and live far off and keep them up-to-date on the progression of his health. These are the first people you need to contact when your LO passes away so they can make travel arrangements immediately. Do you want to have an evening or morning service (consider the weather)? Do you want to hold the service on a weekend? If so, which day? A Saturday or a Sunday?

Most funeral homes charge an extra fee (and it can be exorbitant!) if the funeral is put off too long, for refrigeration, so make sure you discuss this with the funeral director if you know ahead of time that you will have to wait for out-of-town friends or family.

Don't be rushed if his wishes are to be cremated with no viewing. The funeral or service can be put off for months if need be in that case. However, if there is to be a viewing followed by cremation, you will have to have a service rather quickly unless you don't mind paying the extra refrigeration fees.

Funeral Reception

Where is the reception to be held? Don't try to do everything all by yourself. If someone volunteers, take them up on the offer. Put someone in charge of the food.

Florist

Friends & family will want a suggestion for where to order the flowers from. Have a florist selected in advance with contact information ready.

Agenda

Work with the funeral director in regard to the order of the funeral. When it is complete, type it up, make several copies and place the plans in a separate folder for later.

What to provide the Funeral Director when making funeral arrangements

- Full name of your LO
- Occupation
- Date of birth

- Place of birth
- Social security number
- Residence address
- Spouse's name (maiden name)
- Father's name, mother's maiden name
- Place of burial or disposition
- Discharge paper, if he is a veteran

What to provide the Funeral Director with after your LO dies

- The agenda
- The death certificate
- The music plans and the actual tape if there is one
- The florist of choice
- Clothing – including underclothing. Shoes are optional.
- A recent photograph
- A list of the Pallbearer's names
- Data for the obituary- clubs, organizations, honors
- If Memorial Contributions are desired, organize names.
- Insurance policies that they might assist with claims, if so desired.
- Instructions on how the body is to be treated: glasses, dentures, make-up, hair.

- The person who will be officiating; his contact information
- The time and day you have available to meet with him/her to go over all final plans for the funeral. You will have already gone over most of it with him/her after you received the diagnosis as suggested in the earlier part of this chapter.

Funeral services (if applicable) include:

- Coordination with clergy, cemetery or crematory
- Coordination of shipping details
- Assistance with the Veterans Administration claim
- Notification to Social Security Administration
- Obtaining certified copies of death certificate
- Preparing of obituary notices for newspapers
- Assistance with insurance claims

Other services or merchandise funeral homes can provide:

- Clothing
- Flowers
- Memorial Folders or prayer cards
- Special music

- A picture of your LO in the form of a plaque with the background of your choice and a poem or song
- Pre-arranged funeral plans

Try and involve your LO in as much of the planning as he desires. Be sure to have him sign the paper that the plans have been written on so no one can say later that you aren't following his wishes. For the remainder of the plans, involve your family. With the proper planning, it will be organized, less hectic and bring peace instead of chaos.

Thank you cards

Make your address labels for thank you cards. The funeral home usually supplies these cards. Some of these must be addressed after his passing. Example:

- The hospice agency
- The funeral director and funeral home
- The soloist/organist
- The clergy who officiates
- The pallbearers
- Those who sent flowers
- Those who hosted the reception
- Those who brought food
- Those who attended

Chapter Four

Preparing for Death at Home

The initial shock to your system has passed and now it's time to get to work. You will still be in the grief process for quite some time but staying busy and working your plan will help you psychologically.

If your LO has been growing weaker physically, he may qualify for hospice. (This chapter is written with the totally dependent LO in mind)

You need to discuss allowing hospice to come into your home to perform the homecare with your loved one. If he agrees, call the hospice of your choice and ask for a social worker to come over to talk to both of you about their services. If you feel other family members may want to be included at this point, invite them for the meeting. (See chapter 4 for more on hospice definitions)

When it gets close to the end, you must be prepared for a good number of visitors to be coming through your home on a regular basis when you care for your dying LO. You must use common sense in regard to the number of visitors allowed per day. Be aware of how tired your LO gets from these visits. Family and friends often get so wrapped up in their own needs and grief that they don't realize the toll they are taking on the hospice patient. It will be up to you to set boundaries.

The length of the visit is just as important to monitor. Many of the people who come to visit have not seen your LO for a while so will tend to overstay their welcome. If you aren't vigilant, every day can turn into a party, you foot the bill and your LO can become easily exhausted. Keep in mind that you are being depended on for every detail, so you do not have the luxury of the visit. Rather, you have the sole responsibility of the care.

Getting the House Ready

The following is a checklist for you to look over. You may want to implement some or all of the following suggestions in your home.

- Have some folding chairs on hand for visitors. The smaller, the better.

- Stock your freezer with some frozen, tasty entrees such as lasagna, deep dish pot pie etc. When you have a good size group, it's easy to pop them in the oven so the visitors don't have to go out or you don't feel you have to cook at an inopportune time.

- Have a couple of folding TV tray sets available for your guests.

- Set up a small table in your LO's room on which to place the following care essentials: a box of Latex gloves, Kleenex, a roll of paper towels, mouth moisturizer, toothettes, a stack of paper cups, a pitcher of cold water, moisture barrier ointment, peri-wash spray, a roll of small trash bags, cornstarch powder, room deodorizer, a stack of paper bed pads, his weekly medicine container and Eucerin lotion.

- If your LO enjoys a particular kind of music, see to it that you acquire it for him. The cable service has a block of about 100 different types of music, commercial free that you can purchase by the month.

- A scented candle or incense adds a nice touch if you think your LO would like that.

- Keep a lined, covered waste paper container in his room. We place most all trash in ours expect for soiled diapers and paper bed pads. We take those out immediately because of odor.

- You should also keep a few over the counter medications handy if he is not on hospice. Nausea suppositories, a fever and pain reducer, throat lozenges and cough medicine. If he is on hospice, they will provide these in addition to his other medications relevant to his condition.

- If space permits and you want to constantly be at his side, get a folding cot (if there is no other bed in his room) that you can sleep on at night and take back out in the morning.

- If you are going to sleep in your own room, get a baby monitor and leave it on at night so you can hear him if he calls. They usually come with a belt-clip portable unit you can connect to your clothing during the day when you are busy in other parts of the house or in the yard.

- Mount a clock on his wall directly above where he is lying. Make sure it has a second hand. You or the nurse will use this when you need to time his pulse and respirations later.

- If he is on oxygen, the room can get very hot from the concentrator. We usually plug the unit into the outlet closest to the door so that we can "park" the machine outside the bedroom. This will make the room much cooler for your LO. If he starts getting fever, then this comfort measure becomes even more important.

- If your LO is incontinent and does not wear a catheter, make sure you are consistent in checking him for diaper changes. Keep plenty of supplies on hand for him.

- Make sure that you keep a close eye on his medication and reorder in advance so you don't run out. His pain medication is of the utmost in importance right now to keep him comfortable.

- Prepare a fact sheet on your LO with the following information listed, make three copies for those who ask for it and place it in a folder; put it in his room in a drawer so that you can easily locate it when the time comes or post it on the wall:

Fact Sheet List

- **Patients' name**
- **Date of birth and age**
- **Address**
- **Your phone number and relationship to your LO**

- **A list of all of his current medications**
- **The name of the hospice agency, their phone number and your nurses' name**
- **Your LO's doctors' name and phone number**
- **The time you last saw him alive (you can fill this in after he passes away, of course)**
- **His diagnosis**

These are some of the mechanics in caregiving but nothing means more to your LO than the tender loving words and touches you can provide better than anyone in his life right now. This death belongs to the two of you, for the most part, and will be what you make of it.

With prayer, a little organization and a whole lot of love, you will more than get through this- you will be proud of yourself and your LO will appreciate it more than he can voice right now.

Chapter Five
Coping with the Flood of Mixed Emotions

There are many books written on caregiving and most of them address at least part of a chapter on the emotional responses of the patient. However, I have yet to see anyone focus exclusively on the family caregiver with the exception of caregiver burn-out.

In this chapter I will attempt to identify the emotions you, the family caregiver, may be experiencing. Then I will help you to resolve them. It's up to you to use this emotional prescription or not.

Denial:

(When you or a family member other than the terminally ill LO is in denial) "Everything is going to be all right. He really isn't as sick as they say he is. All I have to do is take real good care of him, get him on vitamins, get him off the drugs, see to it that he eats nutritional food and he will get well. Most doctors don't know what they're doing anyway. There has to be another explanation for what's happening and I'm going to find it. I am going to make him exercise every day and maybe a little therapy wouldn't hurt. He has to try harder. I'm not going to let him give up and just die! If he thinks I'm going to stand by and allow him to stay in bed and wither away, he's got another thing coming. We are going to start a new daily regimen. He has to fight the pain and I don't want to hear him complaining about pain. If we give in to it, it will be over and that just can't happen. If we try hard enough, we can whip this thing."

Or (when it's your LO in denial) "The doctor has made a terrible mistake. The tests must have gotten mixed up and he is misreading the symptoms. They have to mean that I am sick with something else and he just doesn't know. I'm not going to tell my family or friends what he said or they will give up on me and without the support I need, I will die. I have to keep this to myself and start taking better care of myself. I'll go see another doctor and another until I get the report I know is correct; that I am not dying, but have something which can be cured."

RESOLUTION:

Re: You or other family members-

Faith is one thing, denial is another but there is a thin line between the two and it's of the utmost importance that you find that line before you proceed to make your LO miserable. Human beings have an innate drive to stay alive at all costs, so it's natural for you to want to fight this for your LO because you identify. You wouldn't want someone resigning themselves to a report that you were terminally ill. The problem with denial is that as your LO begins to deteriorate, if you have voiced strongly that you aren't accepting the diagnosis, he will be very reluctant to share his fears, his feelings and above all else, his depression.

He doesn't want to anger or disappoint you, especially with all the effort you are exerting in trying to make him get "better". I'm not saying for you to get the shovel, but to remain objective and not to put undue pressure on him by forcing him to perform for you to make YOU feel better. This isn't about you. It's about him, his comfort, his life and, yes, his death.

The Indians used to say of a fallen warrior, "It was a good death" to describe bravery and determination. You have the privilege and have taken on the responsibility to help your LO have a good death. One that is filled with peace instead of fear; closure instead of unresolved issues and emotions.

What does he want to do? Who does he want to see? Where does he want to go? Start taking notes and enlist the assistance of your family to help him achieve his goals. Don't waste this precious time trying to convince him that he is not going to die. Instead, make the most of every minute you have left with him to be his eyes, ears and legs. Later on you will have to speak for him in anticipation of his wishes when he can no longer speak for himself. Get to know him better than you do now.

Re: your LO

Sometimes when someone learns he is going to die soon, he will overtax himself trying to prove that he isn't to his detriment. His health may begin to decline faster and in many cases, his pain increases. Then he becomes angry with himself or with those closest to him. If you are the primary caregiver, that means you.

How do you lovingly communicate to him that you aren't giving up on him when you tell him to pace himself? You say something like "Dad, I am standing with you and admire your resolve to get well but we don't have to do everything in one day. Let's take it a bit slower so we can get more done in the long run. You need to consider my health too. You're wearing me out!"

It won't hurt at first for you to allow this mindset without trying to convince him that he is terminally ill, if he is still able to do some things for himself. Let him talk about his position without your debating the subject. He might not want to talk about it. Instead, you may simply notice that he is pursuing life more aggressively and may not even want anyone else in the family to know. Respect this area of his control right now.

If he has dementia, you don't have to talk about it at all. There is no need to. There won't be any denial either.

Anger:

"I am angry with my LO. He should have taken better care of himself. We kept telling him to go to the doctor and he just wouldn't listen. He says he loves us but if he really did, he would have seen the doctor when we told him to."

Or "I am angry with the doctor. They should have known this was coming. They don't care about their patients- they have so many patients that it doesn't matter to them if they lose one."

Or "I am angry at my family. Where were they when I had to take Dad to the doctor and got the bad news? Where was my support system? They haven't had time to visit- too busy with their own careers and families. What about mine? No one thinks about what I am going through. They won't even help out financially but they are all ready to make me account for every dime I need to spend out of Dad's money for his needs."

RESOLUTION:

Re: Your LO-

Anger is a cancer that will eat away at you and right now you don't have the time to indulge yourself. First of all, it's not your LO's choice to be sick and this is what you have to deal with right now. What good can possibly come from being angry with him? Do you think it will make you feel good? Will it make him "snap", do ya think? This is the end of his life. No time for teaching him a lesson so he will behave next time. There won't be a next time. All there is, is now so forgive him and allow compassion to well up within you and reach out to him. It's not up to you to punish him with neglect or the silent treatment. Maybe he blew it due to unhealthy choices (unless he has dementia), but so have all of us at least a few times during our lifetime.

Re: The doctor-

Your time with your LO is precious right now. Don't waste one single emotional moment on being angry with the doctor. You aren't going to change the entire medical profession. He may redeem himself with you if you keep your cool and allow him to continue helping you with your LO. You will also need the doctor's recommendation for hospice care so don't alienate him. Don't burn any bridges or close any doors.

Re: Family members-

You are evidently the most trusted and valuable person in your family. You are also the most blessed. Think about it. You are the one adult child who will be able to share your LO's final days with him. What a privilege! What a sweet time together. You will be privy to see the real person who may have been hiding behind a facade of a lifetime of pride.

When a person learns he is going to die, that big front they have put up around others comes crumbling down and all that is left is the honest review of their lifetime. They usually want to make peace with all they have offended and forgive those who have offended them. You aren't the one in that bed but you can learn from him and forgive right now instead of waiting until you are.

Fear:

"I am afraid of being alone. He has always been here for me and I can't imagine living without him to take care of anymore. I've been doing this for so long. How will I fill my time?"

Or "I am afraid I won't be able to do this right? I'm not a medical professional and this is serious. What if I mess up and fail? I can't possibly do for him what the hospital can do. But he said he didn't want to die in the hospital so how can I ask him to go?"

RESOLUTION:

Re: Being alone-

Call your doctor and see if your LO qualifies for hospice. If he does, you will be inundated with a patient/family support system immediately. There is no waiting period. Whenever we have called for one of our patients and they were approved, the next day hospice came to do the evaluation and the day after that the team members began calling to set up appointments with us. (Chapter Eight will describe the function of hospice)

If he does not qualify for hospice yet, ask your doctor for a referral for a home health agency. They will provide many of the same services that hospice does and then when your LO has less than 6 months to live, you can ask your doctor to sign the referral to a hospice and service can be transferred.

Re: Your adequacy as a care-giver-

For centuries there were no hospitals, nursing homes or other medical facilities to house patients and family cared for their own dying relatives. No one gave a thought as to their ability to do so. There is no "right."

All there is, is your ability to love your LO right now. You will have plenty of guidance every step of the way.

At home, you and the family will have more access to your LO. At home, there are no needles and constant blinking lights and a parade of nurses coming in day and night to disturb him. What can a hospital do for him now? He is terminally ill- they can't save his life. His pain can be managed very effectively at home and you will be doing the most loving act he has ever received over his entire life.

4. Guilt:

"I feel guilty because I want my LO to die. He wouldn't want to go on like this and I have a very hard time seeing him waste away. I can't tell anyone how I feel because they would think I was cruel and cold to say such a thing."

Or "I feel guilty now that my Dad has dementia, is bed-bound and close to death because I mistreated him. I actually wrestled with him and hit him on more than one occasion when I got frustrated. I could never tell anyone about this but I don't know how to get over this guilt. I am so sorry and feel now it's too late to make it up to him. I now realize that he didn't know what he was doing."

RESOLUTION:

Re: Wanting him to die-

I know this may sound strange, but if you didn't love him, you wouldn't care if he died or not. It wouldn't matter to you that he was in pain if you didn't care. The vast majority of family caregivers feel exactly the same way. They just want it over for their LO. Especially when they know it's inevitable. You just don't want to see someone you love suffer. You don't want to see your relatives in pain either.

Start praying to the Lord to take him and just make him as comfortable as possible. Talk to your pastor and/or ask for the hospice chaplain to come by for a visit. Tell them your feelings. They will pray with you. Forgive yourself. It's painful to watch someone you love die. It's only natural to want it over quickly.

Re: Elderly abuse

It's unfortunate that you mistreated your LO, but now that you realize how wrong you were, you have a chance to make it up to him by giving him the love and attention he so desperately needs.

You have to be honest with yourself though. If you ever start to feel that you are losing control again, you owe it to you LO and yourself to look for an alternate living facility. Ask his doctor or social worker to recommend a place that specializes in terminally ill patients.

Ask his forgiveness even if you don't think he will understand you and don't expect a response. He might not be able to adequately process your intentions.

Then, ask God's forgiveness because you have dishonored your parent. Things will start going well for you again when you have repented and received His forgiveness according to His Word, and He forgives immediately. Put the past behind you, stop feeling guilty and get on with making this the sweetest time you have ever had with your LO.

There are many more emotions you may be feeling, but these are the most destructive and that's why I have dealt with them.

Focus on your LO's care and the love he needs you to express to him. That's the most important step you can take right now to speed the healing of your own emotions so you can help him with his.

When Your Loved One is Angry or Paranoid

Although this chapter had to do with the family's emotions, I thought it would be helpful to include some additional information on the dementia patients' anger and paranoia.

The most important fact you will need to accept when caring for a dementia victim who leans toward an angry behavior pattern is that they truly have **no control** over their actions or the way they express their feelings. It may be very difficult for you to accept this mindset.

If your LO was usually angry when his mind was well, you may feel he is just being extra mean and stubborn now. You may only detect a small change at first and believe he is acting this way on purpose and could control his temper if given the proper incentive. You may try and lay a guilt **trip** on him, to no avail.

If he was normally pleasant before and now it seems his personality has changed, you may feel mixed emotions in your new perception of him. If a doctor has informed you that he does indeed have dementia, then you must accept that you are dealing with an entirely different person who desperately needs your patience and kindness.

Listed on the following pages are some distraction techniques and ideas which have worked for us in the past. Keep trying the different methods until you have successfully tasted sweet victory and you will be proud of yourself. Whatever you do, don't react in anger or you will compound the problem and then feel guilty when all is said and done.

Tip # 1:

Above all, don't argue or debate with your LO. You can't possibly win. Now, you will really want to, especially if you're caring for a parent who always had the last word, got his way and disregarded your opinions and feelings when you were young and too little and helpless to assert yourself. You may feel that you have the upper hand now that he is the helpless one and that it's payback time. Please understand this- if you are considering going this route, it borders on abuse. Try and bring peace through forgiving him. After all, how much satisfaction can there possibly be in winning a senseless argument with a mentally and physically challenged helpless individual anyway? Your own self image will go in the dunker very quickly if you behave immaturely and lash out at your LO. Rationalize your acts of patience and kindness by telling yourself that your LO won't remember how brilliantly you debated with him in 5 minutes anyway! That will give you pause.

Tip # 2:

Entice your LO into another room or to go with you outside, if weather permits. If he is wheelchair bound, this can be fairly easy. If he is ambulatory it may require a little more persuading so do yourself a favor and smile as you speak softly, make the suggestion and take him gently by the hand if he will allow it. Sometimes a change of scenery is all that's needed to turn his mood around. He will usually forget he was angry.

Tip # 3:

Don't laugh at this one until you try it- it really works! **Change your clothes and or hair** and then walk back into the room and say something like "Well, hello! How have you been?" In other words, start over again. The changes will often times cause him to forget that it was you his anger was directed toward. We keep a couple of nurses' smocks on hand and a stethoscope to hang around our necks so we can "check them out." Even the most obstinate person will respect "the uniform."

Tip # 4:

As soon as the conversation gets hot, head for the freezer. We keep emergency bowls of ice cream made up for such times. Our motto is "Ice cream makes the world go round." Once you present him with a sweet treat, he will completely forget he was ever upset at all and make sure you don't remind him! If his passion is candy, pie, or whatever it is, keep it close by and serve it right up to alter his mood.

Tip # 5:

Eliminate all noise within his earshot if possible. Noise can bring on catastrophic reactions faster than any other outside stimuli. If you are in the living room and the TV or radio is on very loud and there are several family members talking, laughing or arguing, it can really set someone with dementia off. Remember, his brain can't filter out the overload to the senses as a well-minded person can. He can become confused when he can't process what is going on. Take him to a quiet room, free from all movement, bright lights and noise and then slowly and quietly sit with him until he is calm. If he will allow you to, stroke his hair and tell him how much you love him. Speak softly and remember to smile. Speak in no more than five word sentences and get at his eye level and above all, remember to smile. **Don't** question him.

Tip # 6:

Many angry reactions can be prevented by simply explaining what you are doing before

working with your LO. For example: if he gets angry at bath time, ask yourself if you are jerking him around roughly and not taking time to explain **each step** of the process as you go. Tell him "I am going to help you bathe. Now I am going to take your shirt off. Now let's take off your pants." and "I am going to put water on your hair to wash it." Make sure he remains covered by a towel as you bathe different parts of his body. This way he still keeps his dignity, doesn't feel molested or give you an argument. Don't assume that he should know the routine by now and that he doesn't need any warning as to the steps of the process. He needs to be told each and every time. His memory is no where near like yours is. Treat him as such.

Tip # 7:

Don't rush him. Take your time to move in slow motion. To move at a normal pace can be devastating to him. Again, I can't say it enough: speak softly and slowly in five words or less sentences.

Tip # 8:

Don't expect him to do anything if he is tired or not feeling well that day. We don't like to be forced to do even the simplest tasks when we feel bad. He has lost all social awareness and he wears his heart on his sleeves- he has a lack of self control and will physically and /or verbally let you know if you are displeasing him. His emotions are greatly amplified above yours and are extremely sensitive.

Tip # 9:

Don't overload him with instructions. If he has to think of too many things at the same time and remember how to do them, regardless of how easy they seem to you, he can get frustrated and lash out at you as an act of self defense. Lead him one step at a time in short sentences, speaking softly and smiling all the while, telling him what you want him to do. When he completes one step then slowly move to the next and be sure to praise him!

Tip # 10:

How about just leaving him alone? What a novel idea! Give him his space. If you are trying to get him ready to go somewhere or to take a bath, wait 10 minutes and then try it again. OR, you could try having another family member take a shot at it. Above all, express your love in words, by touch and by your facial expressions. Mercy, grace, forgiveness and love are the most effective ways to handle anger and will quench even the most fierce, raging fire within your LO.

Chapter Six

Medical Problems of the Bed Bound Person

If your terminally ill loved one has declined to the point that he is bed bound, there are precautions you must take to keep him as comfortable as possible. I'm going to list below a few of the more common problems that families face when caring for their loved ones at home and tip to dealing with them.

Dementia

Entire books have been written on dementia, so I'm not going to attempt anything in these two pages but to identify some of the symptoms of the malady. If you notice that your LO is exhibiting a combination of these symptoms, contact his doctor and make an appointment.

There are many types of dementia, the most common being Alzheimer's disease.

Just because a person begins to get a little forgetful as he gets older, doesn't necessarily mean he is getting Alzheimer's. There is more than one symptom involved in the diagnosis that a doctor, usually a neurologist, makes

The following is a list of some of these symptoms:

Symptoms of dementia

1. Memory problems
2. Word-finding problems
3. Paranoia
4. Loss of coordination
5. Loss of a sense of time
6. Confusion
7. Loss of interest in appearance & hygiene
8. Depression
9. Loss of ability to make decisions
10. Vision problems
11. Personality changes
12. Preference changes
13. The person becomes a danger to himself
14. Sleep patterns change
15. Weight loss
16. Incontinence
17. Balance problems

Constipation & Diarrhea

Once upon a time, long ago, someone started an urban legend that if the elderly didn't take boatloads of laxatives daily, they would become so clogged up that they would explode. They all seemed to buy it. That's why if your LO misses a bowel movement for one day, he panics and downs the laxatives.

Unfortunately, this causes constipation. When someone habitually takes laxatives to move their bowels, his body comes to rely on them, gets lazy and ceases to function naturally.

It's easier for a family caregiver to give in to their LO and give him his laxatives than to put up with his complaining, but it's not healthy for him if they take them out of habit rather than true constipation.

When someone, regardless of his age, gets constipated, it can be very painful. Hemorrhoids can develop quickly and the burning and itching that comes along with the pain can create fear. Anyone who has experienced this can relate and be sympathetic.

Constipation can be caused by a wide variety of conditions. Certain medications, hormonal problems, a lack of water and dietary habits can be the underlying culprits. You need to check the side effects on the information sheet that comes with your LO's medications from the pharmacy. If constipation is one of them, ask his doctor for an alternative.

Invest in a book on a high fiber diet and begin to slowly change your LO's eating habits. Make sure he drinks eight glasses of water daily and don't allow him to eat foods, like cheese, that are known to cause constipation.

Diarrhea can be just as uncomfortable. If your LO has it for longer than a week or it seems to be chronic, they could become dehydrated. If this happens, talk to his doctor. He will probably prescribe some medication to stop the loose bowels but stay on top of it. If he doesn't seem to be getting any better after one day, call the doctor back and see if he can be seen immediately.

The doctor might want to run some tests on him because diarrhea can be a symptom of a major health problem such as colon cancer, impaction or diabetes.

If your LO is lactose intolerant and he gets a hold of a dairy product such as milk, cheese or cream, he could become very ill and diarrhea could start within an hour of ingestion.

If your LO wears adult briefs and has diarrhea, make sure you change him as soon as he has a movement or he will get chapped from the acid and impurities in the feces. Also, use A&D Ointment on his anus to prevent soreness.

Medications

Even if your LO does not have dementia, he still needs help taking his medication if you are having to take care of him.

If he is taking many meds each day and a new one has just been prescribed, ask his doctor or the pharmacist to review the compatibility of all medications involved. Many times there are side effects when the chemical components in different drugs collide such as dizziness, constipation, confusion, agitation, tremors, insomnia and drowsiness. If you notice any unusual behavior in your LO, call his doctor immediately.

You can purchase a small plastic container with built-in compartments for each day of the week, four times a day, to fill with your LO's medications so you can keep track of them easier. Taking this measure can prevent a disastrous episode of double-dosing which could prove to be fatal. We get the "Medi-Set" brand available at most pharmacies. If you fill them weekly, it will take the memory element out of it-even for you!

Don't leave his pill bottles lying around. After you have filled his medication container, place the bottles in a zip-lock bag and put it away so no one can get to it.

Overmedicating is a major problem with the elderly, especially for those who have dementia. It can take many attempts at trying different behavior-modifying medications and dosages before a doctor finds one that works. As your LO's primary caregiver, it will be your responsibility to watch out for side effects and to use common sense when administering his medications.

It's equally important that you stay on top of getting your LO in to see his physician for regular check-ups. He may require a different dosage and/or medication or combination to treat his current condition.

If your LO has had no problem in the past with incontinence, begins a new medication or different dosage of a same medication and begins to have "accidents", tell his doctor about it. It could be the medicine. The elderly have the same delicate balance as a baby and it can be upset by even the smallest change. Don't let too much time go by before you call him. If you wait too long, the incontinence could become irreversible and introduce a new problem that could have otherwise been prevented.

Even over-the-counter medications can present a problem. Always ask the pharmacist before introducing something new to his system. When you talk to him, be sure to go prepared. Provide him with a list of your LO's current medications so he can make an assessment.

When the instructions on the bottle say to take the pills with food, comply. If you don't, it could cause your LO to vomit or worse.

Certain meds are to be taken in the a.m. and others in the evening. Always follow instructions to the letter.

Invest in a pill crusher and a pill splitter. If your LO feels uncomfortable taking a whole pill, try crushing it and putting the powder in his food. Do what works for you.

Pneumonia & Other Breathing Problems

When people of any age and with any medical problem become bed-bound, they are prime candidates for breathing disorders. The angle at which they are lying, combined with the lack of movement, can cause a lung infection because of bacteria. Everyday, ordinary motion keeps all of us healthy, so when we become sedentary, it can reverse our state of health very quickly.

It's bad enough not to be able to breathe but when someone with dementia develops complications in this area, they become totally disoriented, more confused, may stop eating and drinking altogether and can become practically comatose. Their system is so very delicate and fragile that any slight imbalance can throw them off completely.

Also, contrary to popular belief, people don't die of Alzheimer Disease or any other type of dementia. They die from medical complications which arise from dementia. Pneumonia is one of them.

In the latter stages of dementia, people become bed-bound and unless their caregiver sees to it that they are turned from side to side, mucous, and other liquids, can settle in their lungs and cause an infection.

Dementia affects the brain, which in turn can affect our swallowing mechanism. When this happens, anything that is swallowed may not always go into their stomach. It may go into his lungs instead. Once a foreign object enters the lungs, the body tries to rid itself of it by coughing it up. If they are too weak to cough, it can result in volumes of phlegm going into the lungs.

If a liquid continues going into the lungs, it can cause your LO to develop pneumonia.

Pneumonia is characterized by fever, coughing and difficulty breathing. It can be treated by the aggressive use of antibiotics and diuretics to help dry the fluid out of the lungs, and the pushing of fluids, so as to prevent dehydration. If his saturation level is too low, the doctor may order oxygen therapy.

If your LO develops swallowing problems and chokes on liquids, try using a liquid thickener such as "Thickett". This non-flavored powder can be used in any beverage to make it easier to swallow.

When a person gets pneumonia, it can cause them to become very confused and/or non-verbal.

If you suspect your LO has pneumonia, try to keep his head elevated, give him a very small amount of water at a time unless he chokes, and if he does, cease the fluids. Call the doctor or his nurse immediately.

Pain

When your LO complains of pain, ask him the following questions:

1. Where is the pain located?
2. Does the pain throb consistently or does it feel like sharp, knife-like jabs?
3. On a scale of 1-10, 1 being the least and 10 being the most severe, where is your pain?

When you call his doctor or nurse, be ready to answer their questions. They will most likely ask if he has fever, when the last bowel movement was, what medications is he on currently, if he is in pain, crying, dizzy or vomiting. Then tell them the specifics regarding the pain itself based on your LO's answers when you asked him the above questions.

If your LO is ambulatory, the doctor will want to see him in his office, so set up an immediate appointment.

If your LO has home health, the nurse should be notified immediately and she will come right away. After an evaluation, she will consult with the doctor, usually right from your home by phone and he will order the appropriate medication for him.

One of the most common concerns that we have seen family members have regarding pain medication, is that their LO will become addicted to it. If their LO is terminally ill, what does it matter? All that matters is that they are comfortable and not suffering.

Another worry is that their LO is sleeping too much. If the only way your dying LO can be free from pain is to sleep right now, how can you deny him the dosage which will take the torment away?

If your LO does not have dementia and is experiencing considerable pain, you should still ask yourself the above questions.

We aren't saying that overmedicating isn't a problem but what good does it do them to be fully awake and in excruciating pain?

There can be many reasons for a person to have pain and so it really takes a professional to make that determination.

Don't allow your opinions or pride to stand in the way of your LO's relief. Get him the help he is depending on for you to provide as his caregiver.

Pressure Sores

A pressure sore is an open wound on the skin which occurs as a result of prolonged and constant body weight in one specific area of the body. In severe cases, it can become infected and the skin breaks down. In some cases, to the point of rotting away to the bone beneath.

Pressure sores can happen when a person is confined, due to medical reasons, to a chair or a bed. When the person gets close to death, it doesn't matter how often you turn them, they can still appear because the skin cells are no longer receiving, or acting on, the repair messages that the brain is sending.

Below are listed some preventative measures you can take to prevent this very painful condition:

1. Check the mattress to make sure it's not too hard. Hospital beds come with a non-removable plastic cover on their mattress which becomes hardened over time. Unless someone has an open bedsore, they won't qualify for a gel-pad or air-pressure mattress under Medicare guidelines if they do not have hospice service.
2. If your LO does have an open wound, call his nurse or doctor to report it and ask them to order a special mattress for him. If he has home health care or is on hospice, the nurse will come over, assess the situation and ask the doctor to place the order.
3. Sheepskin heel and elbow protectors should be worn to prevent pressure sores. Your home health

agency, hospice agency or local pharmacy will have these in stock.

4. Turn your LO over (if he can't move around by himself) every 2-4 hours. Place a pillow between his legs, ankles, and behind his back when he is on his side. When on his back, be sure to elevate his head to keep the pressure off his tailbone.
5. Keep his skin clean and dry. Gently rub out red areas with a moisture barrier ointment when first observed.
6. Twice to three times daily, massage his entire body with massage lotion or baby oil to stimulate circulation.
7. Call the doctor or nurse as soon as you notice any redness developing. This is a sign that sores are brewing beneath the surface.
8. If your LO has a catheter, make sure he never lays on it or it could quickly develop into a problem area. That also goes for his hospital bed bars and anything else that is in his bed with a hard surface.

You need to protect your LO in many ways and it may seem like a lot of work, but it's worth doing when you consider the alternative. If your LO develops pressure sores, there will be much more pain and the increased work load to go with it.

Dry Skin

As we get older, our skin loses the ability to re-hydrate itself when it gets dry. The natural oils which are abundant when we are children become scarce.

Dry skin turns into itchy skin which causes people to scratch off any oil that is there leading to even drier skin. Listed below are a few suggestions you might try if your LO suffers with this problem.

1. Don't bathe your LO any more than 3 times a week. Don't make the water too hot otherwise you risk drying the skin out more than it already is. Also, use a moisturizing rather than a deodorant soap. Keep the oil out of the tub for safety reasons, but pour it on and rub it in outside of the bathroom after the bath.
2. Use cotton clothing.
3. Cut some fresh Aloe Vera directly from the plant. Peel it, boil it with a little water and then when it's cool, apply it to the dry skin. Do this twice daily.
4. Use a very soft washcloth to bathe him. If you can get a cloth baby diaper, that would be best.
5. Eucerin lotion (found in most drugstores) is great for dry, itchy skin. Be generous in applying it. It won't leave your LO's skin oily either,

6. Water consumption will begin to re-hydrate his skin as well as flush toxins from his body.
7. If he won't stop scratching, use cortisone cream or calamine lotion.
8. Caffeine will cause the itching to worsen besides not being good for him anyway.
9. If it doesn't let up, take him to a dermatologist or his doctor and have him examined.

Malnutrition & Dehydration

If your LO is terminally ill, his appetite will come and go. The very foods he loved all of his life may suddenly hold no special meaning whatsoever. On the other hand, he may begin to request foods he wouldn't touch before. Illnesses can radically affect our taste for foods. Certain medications have side effects which decrease the appetite.

There will come a time when you cannot get your LO to eat anything. At first, he may ask for a particular meal. Then when you bring it to him, he says he isn't hungry or he didn't ask for that.

If you begin to see a pattern developing here, try preparing the food once and then if he doesn't eat it, giving him a high caloric liquid supplement like Nestles 2.0 which contains 550 calories per can.

you had someone to remind you or do the brushing for you, what would your mouth smell like? Nasty thought, right?

Hopefully, you brush at least twice daily. Your LO requires the same care you do. Not only will his breath stay fresh but you will be eliminating harmful germs that could potentially lead to gum or tongue infection and/or mouth sores if left undone.

Here are a few ways you can approach the mouth care:

- Ideally, the brushing is accomplished easiest in the shower. Whenever you shower him, do it there.

- Let's say that your LO still needs limited assistance with brushing. Have his toothbrush ready with toothpaste already on it, paper cup and towel ready before you take him into the bathroom.

- See if he can still brush effectively (in your opinion). If so, let him. If not, ask him to open his mouth so you can finish up.

- If he is in the latter stages of dementia, cannot perform his own oral care and won't open up for you, simply place a paper cup to his lips. His reflex will be to open up to drink. Then quickly, but carefully, place the toothbrush or toothette inside and commence brushing. A toothette is a round paper stick with a small, flavored sponge attached. Be prepared for him to bite down on it and refuse to let go. If he does, gently pull his chin down until he releases it.

- Don't expect him to rinse and expel if he is in the latter stages of dementia. Allow him to swallow and consider yourself fortunate that you even got inside of his mouth at all!

A note about dentures:

Your LO's mouth still needs the same oral care if he wears dentures. Soak the plates at night or brush and set aside in a cup until the next morning. When brushing the plates, line the bottom of the sink with a washcloth to avoid breakage in case they slip and fall. Brush the gums and tongue just as you would the teeth.

If he stops wearing them, the gums will usually shrink and then, after a while, the dentures won't fit or stay in place as they once did. If this happens and you are both in agreement for him to cease from wearing them, don't panic. Leave the plates out and begin to prepare a soft diet. Examples: mashed or baked potatoes, spinach, Jell-O. pudding, oatmeal, meat loaf, ice cream, grits, pancakes, eggs, pimiento cheese, Vienna sausages or tuna salad sandwiches.

As your LO begins to decline, the wearing of dentures will become much less important to you and to him. Our rule of thumb for bed bound, terminally ill patients, is to do whatever makes them the most comfortable. Don't insist on the dentures toward the end for vanity's sake alone.

Nail care

Keep your LO's fingernails clipped way back and blunt. If he ever gets combative with you, you'll soon find out why! Be very careful not to nick the skin or cause him pain or that may be the one thing he never forgets and he won't allow you to clip them again.

If he is a diabetic, it would better to leave the clipping to his nurse's aide or doctor unless you have successful experience doing it yourself. Even a small nick that draws blood can get infected and lead to gangrene.

Remember that the utmost in precaution must be taken with a diabetic. If you do elect to groom his nails yourself, be sure you use an alcohol spray to sterilize the nail tools, your hands, (before you latex-glove them) and his hands before and after the procedure.

If you must use colored nail polish, use the one minute drying type to avoid a mess. Most of the time, we stick with a clear gloss because if it smudges, you can't see it.

The best time to clean his nails is right after his bath so that it loosens and softens any dirt or food under his nails. This makes it easier to remove.

If feces or anything else gets under his nails and you aren't going to bathe him right away, soak his fingers in warm, soapy water before you attempt to clean them. Use a nail brush to loosen the matter and then proceed with a nail file to finish up. The bacteria and acid in feces can lead to infection and sore nail beds, so never leave the cleaning for later.

The feet are often a neglected part of hygienic care in the elderly. The same precautions should be observed when trimming the toenails as the fingernails.

Usually, the fingernails receive more attention, but all extremities demand great caution when coming in contact with sharp objects. If your LO has corns or calluses in addition to a diabetic condition, be sure to consult with his podiatrist before using over-the-counter products to remove them.

You need to look at his feet every day to make sure there are no sores or open blisters. If you find there are, call the doctor or his nurse immediately so they can advise you.

Bath time

We have spoken to many families who have had monumental problems with getting their LO to bathe or to even allow someone else to bathe them.

People with dementia who are combative seem to be more of a challenge, but even the non-verbal and gentle-natured elderly can turn irate and physical when bath time arrives.

There are diverse opinions among the medical professionals as to the reasons for the aversion to bathing. I'll share our opinions, experiences and solutions with you.

A. Sounds

Keep in mind that sights and sounds can be amplified many times over with those who exhibit dementia. The mere sound of running water may be extremely frightening to him. It could sound like an avalanche about to fall on his head.

Because of the strain, the time factor and the unpleasantness, most family members elect to give their LO a bath only 2-3 times weekly.

Any non-routine activity you ask your LO to participate in can, in their own mind, present danger and a threat to his safety. If he is exposed to these unfamiliar sounds so rarely it can cause a catastrophic reaction such as violent or abusive outbursts.

B. Sights

Most bathrooms come equipped with a mirror. Mirrors can cause a person with dementia great confusion. You must remember that things you take for granted every day loom large and scary to your LO. Your reflection as his caregiver can make him believe there are two of you. To avoid this, keep his back towards the mirror or cover it.

Also, he may believe that a naked person is occupying the same small room as himself and when you proceed to disrobe him he can become alarmed.

He may already have word finding problems or difficulty communicating at all, so all he knows to do is to physically defend himself and may, at times, strike out as best he can to fend off the imagined aggressor.

C. Other Factors

The following are some actions which can present and prevent fear of bathing in your loved one:

1. ***Rushing them*** – be patient, take your time and don't begin a bath unless you have plenty of time to complete it cheerfully.
2. ***Talking loudly*** with a demanding tone in your voice – if he isn't hard of hearing speak softly and in very short sentences and whenever possible, look into his eyes while speaking and always remember to smile. If he does have hearing difficulties, do the above but speak loudly but make sure you don't frown.
3. ***Pulling at his clothes or yanking him around*** – Instead, ask him to help you. For example: When you enter the bathroom, start with a familiar activity like going to the toilet. When you have taken his pants down and he is seated on the toilet, take the opportunity to slip off his shoes, socks and pants. He may object, so say, "I'm going to help you take your bath." He may reply "I don't need/want a bath. I just took one last night (even if he didn't). Whatever you do, DON'T start a debate. You not only won't win, but you'll turn a 30 minute bath into 4 hours trying to win! Stay in motion. You aren't asking his permission, just addressing his concern. Gently proceed disrobing him and talk about his childhood or some subject

that is meaningful to him. Anything to distract him from the unpleasantness of "the dreaded bath"!

How to Bathe an Adult in the Shower

- Try and keep his usual routine as much as possible. Bath time should be planned at the same time and on the same days each week. This way, you will have the least resistance.

- Before you take him to the bathroom, have the bath water ready, or if you are giving him a shower, the water set at the correct temperature. Have all bath supplies (liquid pump soap, washcloth, towels, shampoo, toothbrush with the toothpaste already on it, floor mat, powder and lotion) laid out to make the ritual as easy as possible.

- Never leave him alone in the bathtub. He could change the temperature of the water and burn himself.

- If your LO is very confused and resistant, consider wearing a white nurses uniform. The elderly respect a uniform and the authority that comes with it. As far as he is concerned, you are a doctor or a nurse and have the right to direct him.

- Use a shower bench whether you are giving him a bath or a shower. It can be extremely difficult for both of you to have to get him up and down to the bottom of a tub, especially when he is wet and slippery.

- Use a minimum amount of soap to make the rinsing easier. Avoid using oils in the tub area altogether.

- If he is overweight, make sure you clean any flaps or folds of skin and rinse them well to avoid a rash. When it's time to dry them, apply powder or cornstarch to them to absorb any moisture of the day.

- Regardless of how embarrassing it may be to you to clean his genitals, they must be washed and rinsed thoroughly to avoid rashes and possible sores from forming. If he doesn't qualify for a home health aide and you cannot bring yourself to do this, ask another family member.

- To prevent a disastrous fall, dry all puddles of water immediately. Make sure you dry his hands before he reaches for the grab bars to steady himself upon exiting the tub.

- A terrycloth robe can be extremely beneficial for him to put on immediately after his bath. It helps to keep him warm while you tend to dry the rest of his body.

- Stay on the lookout for agitation if you choose to use a blow dryer on his hair. The noise may upset or frighten him. If you do, make sure you hold it at least 12 inches from his scalp so you don't burn him. Remember, painful memories are among the last to go!

- Use a very large, soft towel to cover him with as you are bathing him to preserve his dignity. Keep in mind how you would feel if you were naked for an extended period of time; helpless and at the mercy of a stranger, which is what you are or will eventually become as the dementia progresses.

- Have him brush his teeth in the bathtub during the shower. This way, it makes less of a mess. We make it very easy for our residents by using battery operated toothbrushes.

How to Bathe a Bed Bound Person

A bed or sponge bath might be more appropriate in certain circumstances. If he can't sit up, is very heavy or semi-conscience, he will require a bed bath. If he gets hysterical in the tub or shower and grows increasingly combative, try a sponge bath but still taking care to leave him covered, exposing only the area you are bathing and keep him warm.

Make sure not to use regular soap as it is very hard to rinse thoroughly. Instead, use a no-rinse soap, available at most medical supply houses and pharmacies. Simply pour the directed amount into a small plastic basin filled with warm water. Use the washcloth to clean him and then dry one area at a time. Change the bath water 3 times: (1) to clean his face and then upper body (2) to clean the back and genital area and (3) to clean his legs and feet.

Bath Time Close to the End of Life

When you have been told that your LO is very close to passing away and/or is having a difficult time breathing or may be experiencing pain, you should not put him through any more discomfort than absolutely necessary. At this point, bathing is no longer necessary, neither is turning him around the clock.

You might want to use a warm cloth to wipe his face and head, but a full bed bath would only be more traumatic than beneficial to him.

When he is in what is called "the active dying process", he will stop voiding urine and feces because he has already stopped taking in fluids and food. Diaper changes will cease. If he does urinate or have a slight bowel movement, be very gentle as you change him. If you notice that any remaining urine is turning dark red, don't be alarmed. It's a normal part of the dying process.

It's not an easy feat; getting over to the other side. Make his last few hours or days on this earth as comfortable as you possibly can.

Chapter Eight
The Role Hospice Plays

The National Hospice Organization has established certain guidelines to help doctors determine if a patient is a candidate for hospice care to be paid by Medicare. One of these conditions is that the patient has less than six months to live. Only your LO's personal doctor can make this determination.

Once he has given his permission, be prepared for an entire team of support to envelope you and your LO in support, compassion and love.

Hospice performs comfort and palliative care only. No life saving measures are taken when a patient is on hospice. In most cases, a do not resuscitate (DNR) order is required before they take on a case. Aggressive treatment such as feeding tubes, ventilators, surgery, radiation or chemotherapy will not be a part of the hospice care plan for your LO.

However, if your LO is having a difficult time breathing, oxygen may be ordered to ease his panic. If he is in pain, they will very effectively manage it so that only in very rare cases will the patient feel any discomfort.

The differences between a regular home health agency and hospice care are as follows:

Hospice cares for terminally ill patients exclusively, therefore, their entire staff is trained specifically to focus on every need of and make provision for the dying patient and their family. Normally, a dying patient will not be dropped from service except in very rare circumstances. They are followed all the way through death by their team.

On the other hand, the home health staff cares for the patient who has just left the hospital and needs help getting back to normal again, usually for a period of 2-4 weeks only.

The admission requirements are very stringent and upheld to the letter. They may also be called in for temporary service for patients who have had a change, at home, in their medication or have a physical need which cannot be addressed by their doctor (because they may be bed-bound) such as a bed sore.

They also care for terminally ill patients but don't specialize in their treatment and their staff is not trained in the care of the dying and their families. They have an important role in the care profession but as far as terminal care goes, hospice is second to none.

Hospice has much more latitude regarding the strongest pain medication permitted in a home setting.

They can provide medication relative to the patient's diagnosis at no charge to the family and more supplies than home health agencies are permitted by Medicare guidelines are, such as diapers, gloves, peri-wash, mouth moisturizer, mouthwash, bed pads, moisture barrier ointment, heel & elbow protectors etc.

Hospice has a registered pharmacist on staff who will come out to your home and assess your LO if he is having a pain management problem or any type of other physical ailment that the nurse has been unable to bring under control. Home health doesn't do this.

Most people think that when hospice comes out to their home, that they will stay 24/7 but this isn't the case. The aide will be assigned 3-5 days a week to do his personal grooming for 45 minutes per visit. They are not sitters.

Now, let's talk about the hospice team members and their functions.

1) The Medical Director (in collaboration with the attending physician): This person comes out to your home and makes the initial examination of your LO and certifies him for hospice care. She then will develop a care plan specifically to fit his needs, develops the team who will be providing care for your LO and write the orders. She will continue to monitor and assess the care plan, evaluate reported symptoms and manage his pain.

2) The Nurse: Your LO will be assigned a nurse who will come at least once a week and in between regularly scheduled visits when necessary. Her official title is "RN Case Manager." The following is a list of the skills and services your hospice nurse provides: (she will…)

- Make a complete initial assessment of your LO's state of health.
- Present the hospice philosophy and the services provided by her agency.
- Explain your LO's rights and responsibilities.
- Assess wishes and expectations for everyone involved and talk over the resources available regarding his care.
- Provide volunteer support for you, your LO and/or your family.
- Teach you or your family how to physically care for your LO.
- Assess pain, pain management's effectiveness and other symptoms.
- Assess blood pressure and all other vital signs including pain.
- Provide comfort measures for pain and other symptom relief.
- Assess cardiovascular, pulmonary and respiratory status.

- Teach you symptom control and relief measures.
- Teach you how many liters of oxygen your LO needs.
- Teach you how to give medications to your LO, identify need for change, addition or other plan or dose adjustment.
- Teach effective oral care for your LO.
- Observe each week if there is the presence or signs of infection.
- Teach you and your family about realistic expectations of the disease process.
- Teach all involved the signs and symptoms of impending death.
- Teach you how to suction your LO safely.
- How to transfer your LO safely.
- Assess if choking and aspiration are going on and instruct you on what to do to help your LO.
- Teach you on safe eating measures.
- Assess mental status and sleep disturbances.
- Provide you and your family emotional support.
- Teach you how to turn your loved one safely

- Teach you how to change the dressings for your LO's bed sores and how to watch for infection.
- Check for and remove impactions.
- Change catheter as needed.
- Teach you daily catheter care.
- Monitor bowel patterns.
- Counsel you regarding your LO's hydration, diet and nutrition.
- Explain the changes you should expect as your LO continues to decline.

She will confer with the hospice physician and develop a care plan in concert with the other hospice team members and order any medical equipment he needs.

She will take his vital signs; blood pressure, temperature, pulse and number of respirations and then record them on a report she will then leave a folder in his room. If he has any wounds, she will dress them. If he needs medication, she will order them and they will be delivered to your home that same day. She will closely follow his symptoms to see if there are any side effects to the medication and then make adjustments if need be.

If he is in pain, has fever, is having difficulty breathing or has any other medical need, she will contact the hospice doctor assigned to his case and receive instructions directly from him. She will also consult with you, give you care instructions and get your opinion on his care plan.

3) The Home Health Aide or Certified Nursing Assistant: This person is not a nurse but has been certified to do the following:

- Give your LO his bath (bed or tub).
- Clean his mouth and teeth and/or dentures.
- Apply lotion, moisture barrier ointment and powder.
- Change his clothes and diapers and his bedclothes.
- Shave him.
- Straighten up his room,
- Take out his trash and place his soiled laundry where you want her to.
- Observe your LO's condition and report back to the team manager.
- Safely transfer your LO.

- Provide respite care.
- Prepare meals.
- Provide homemaker services.
- Provide comfort care.

She will be assigned to come out 45 minutes to an hour, 3-5 times weekly, depending on the nurse's recommendation and the hospice doctor's decision based on your LO's need.

She is not responsible for taking vitals or anything else that the nurse handles. She will report any change in your LO's condition in writing to the agency, and by phone if she feels the situation needs immediate attention.

4) The Social Worker: This team member serves an invaluable purpose in the lives of the terminally ill patient and his family. She assesses the needs of each individual involved and finds ways to provide for them through referral methods to other community resources. She will make herself available to your entire family as a compassionate counselor. She will schedule regular weekly visits to see your LO at your convenience. The following is a list of her role in your LO's care:

- Funeral & burial assistance

- Provide you and your family with information regarding food acquisition, costs of needed medication and other community resources which will enable your LO to remain in the home.

- Grief counseling and support

- Depression/fear assessed and addressed

5) The Chaplain or other spiritual counselor: This spiritual advisor makes himself available to pray with and counsel the patient and his entire family as needed, and is always mindful of their particular beliefs and faith. He will schedule a weekly visit to see your LO. The family comes to rely on his gentle guidance and advice. Listed below are his responsibilities to you, your LO and your family:

- Spiritual assessment and care
- Prayer with you, your LO and all family members involved
- Listening, support and availability
- Participation in your LO's sacred or spiritual practices and rituals

- Funeral & burial assistance

6) **The Hospice Volunteer:** These amazing people have no motive for the heartfelt work they do. Just look at what services they provide without pay:

- Comfort, friendship and companionship
- Errands & transportation
- Comfort & dignity maintained/provided for you, your LO and your family

7) **Dietician/Nutritional counseling:**
   - Assesses your LO when he has decreased intake, weight loss, or nausea
   - Assists with swallowing difficulties
   - Advises on nutritional supplements and snacks to increase protein and caloric intake
   - Evaluation of nutritional deficits and needs

8) **Occupational Therapist:**
   - Evaluation of how well your LO can move around to help himself
   - If you need any special medical equipment or assistive devices, she can get them ordered for you after an evaluation
   - Assessment of upper body function and strength

9) Physical Therapist:

- Safe transfer training
- Strengthening/exercise program
- Teaches you how to lift safely
- Shows how to administer bed mobility exercises

10) Speech-language pathologist:

- Evaluates your Food texture recommendation
- Suggests alternate communication program
- LO for speech/swallowing problems

11) Massage, art, music or other therapies

Pet therapy

Assessment plan to engage your LO in activities to provide support, enjoyment, quality and dignity

Evaluation and intervention based on you and your LO's unique wishes and needs that support care, comfort and death in the setting of his choice

Will improve muscle tone, sleep, and relaxation with massages

Supplies usually provided by hospice (no charge):

- Adult diapers
- Latex gloves
- Wound care supplies and medication
- Prescription medicine if it relates to the diagnosis
- All toiletries
- Peri/incontinence supplies
- Peg tube feeding supplies (some hospice agencies)
- Medical equipment (hospital bed, wheel chair, shower bench, Hoyer lift and trapeze, oxygen concentrator, nebulizer, gel mattress, gel wheelchair pad etc.)
- Short term in-patient & respite care
- Physician on staff (makes home visits as needed)
- Pharmacist on staff (makes home visits as needed)

All of these services and supplies at no cost to you! As you can see, the work hospice does will be invaluable to you, your LO and your family. If you haven't received the recommendation from his physician yet, call him and ask today.

Chapter Nine
Ten Keys to Avoid Caregiver Burn-out

There is a little story I once heard many years ago about a man we will call Sam, who was a workaholic. He would work day and night and some weeks he didn't take a day off and he did this for years.

One day he had a conversation with Pete, a co-worker, who had just gotten back from a two-week vacation in Hawaii.

When Pete told Sam how refreshed he was and how much fun he had with his wife.

Sam said "I wish I could go to Hawaii. I have always wanted to. I have spent the past eleven years dreaming about the waves, the sand, and the ocean breeze. I think about it all the time I am working."

Pete replied "Then why don't you just go. What's stopping you?"

Sam followed Pete's advice and went to Hawaii two months later with his wife. The third day of his vacation, while he was lounging on the beautiful white-sanded beach, breeze blowing in his hair, the sound and sight of the blue-green translucent waves pounding the shore, what do you think was on his mind? You guessed it; The work he wasn't getting done by sitting there in Hawaii!

We must take time for ourselves if we want to be at our best for our family. I'd like to share our own keys to avoiding burn-out as caregivers for the past seventeen years.

Key # 1: Enlist family & friends help

The most obvious thing to do is to get some help. The most obvious place to look to for help is your own family. Enlist your siblings or your own children, if you have them, and if they are willing to help. If not, ask your friends or neighbors to come and stay with your LO while you go grocery shopping or run your errands.

Investigate medical students at the local colleges. Perhaps they need a place to live-in. Check out their references and be sure to talk to their parents and professors before deciding on one. You can trade room and board for their help sitting with your LO while you get away in addition to getting some help around the house. Be sure to set up the rules and guidelines in a written, signed agreement to avoid future misunderstandings.

Key # 2: Get your rest

For at least thirty minutes a day, rest all of your senses.

In our bedroom, we have the windows darkened by solid insulation which permits no light to enter in. We have a ceiling fan to keep it cool in addition to our central air. We have a very comfortable bed. Without fail, once a day, I make sure someone is available to tend to our patients so I can retreat to our room, lie down and rest my senses. I use earplugs to block out all sound. (don't do this unless someone is there to fill in for you)

On occasion, I am able to get a two hour nap! But even if it's only for thirty minutes, I feel refreshed and ready to go again.

While you rest, clear your mind. When my mind is on overload, I picture a huge, blank movie screen and concentrate to keep it blank. You may have your own method. Whatever works for you is fine!

Key # 3: Hire some help

If financial resources are there, hire a live-in housekeeper. Room and board help to cut down on their weekly pay. Screen them well and check out the last three places they worked to get an idea of their character and skills.

It would be best if you hire someone who has had experience working with the elderly so they aren't stand-off-ish when they need to fill in for you. Make sure that you pay them on time and give them at least one day a week off. If they do not perform well, give them their two weeks notice and start again.

Key # 4: Develop a creative outlet

When family caregivers care for someone who is dying, many times they feel like it's futile because "soon he will be gone and there is nothing that I can do that will be of any lasting value." This is far from the truth. How would you feel when he's gone if you didn't do your utmost best to care for him? You are going to know in your heart, years from now, that you provided him with some of the best loved days of his life and a sense of healthy pride will warm you all over just to remember it. To avoid that feeling of futility, create an outlet for yourself at home. Take the time to do something that you really enjoy doing. If you like to cook, prepare food in large quantities and freeze it for when family and friends will be coming over at the end.

If your LO still enjoys eating, prepare his favorites. Cook for your friends or family in exchange for their coming over to stay so you can get out for a while.

If you like gardening, take your portable baby monitor outside with you and do some planting or re-potting.

If you've long ago abandoned your painting or drawing because of raising the kids or your career took up all of your time, pick it up again. This is a terrific outlet. If you are good at faces and bodies, paint or draw your LO from his last photo before he got sick. Talk about therapeutic!

Maybe you enjoy writing. Keep a diary of your caregiving journey or write that book you've always had in you but didn't have the time to do it.

There are many things you can do to stimulate the creativity God put inside you. You will feel fulfilled when you balance this enormous caregiving responsibility with your own need to express that creative spirit.

Key # 5: Emotional outlets

Did you ever see the movie "Steel Magnolias"? (if you didn't, rent it) Remember in the last scene when Sally Fields was sobbing but then without warning, started laughing uncontrollably at her daughter's funeral. It was so real.

Don't hold back the tears or the laughter. Every day, we find a jillion things to laugh at while caregiving for the terminally ill. We laugh at ourselves; humans are really funny if you stop and think about it! Give yourself permission to have some fun. No one will think you are cold or calloused because you don't get up every day and put on sackcloth and ashes. If they do then that's their problem- don't make it yours.

When you feel like crying, cry. If you feel the need to have someone hold you while you cry, ask them.

How will you know if you are crying "too much"? When minutes of crying turn into hours and then into days and you aren't able to concentrate enough to care for your LO, then you need to seek counseling. Make an appointment to see your pastor and tell him how you are feeling. He will pray with you and help you get through this.

Key # 6: Attend church

Try and get away to go to church. If no one will stay with your LO on Sunday mornings, go on Wednesday nights. See if a family member will go with you. Spiritual support will be the primary key to helping you experience hope for the future.

Key # 7: Volunteer services

If your LO is on hospice or has a home health agency, make an appointment with his social worker to discuss any concerns you may have regarding his care and any volunteer services that might be available to sit for you.

Key # 8: Take care of your own health

Take care of your health.

Eat a well balanced diet.

Go for a morning walk daily. This will get you out of the house and give you a fresh new perspective on life.

Get plenty of sleep at night or if your LO has his days and nights mixed up, sleep during the day while he does.

Watch out for the caffeine trap though. That won't help you. It'll just make you nervous in the long run.

Know yourself well enough to guard your alcohol intake. It's not that difficult for you to go from having a drink occasionally to having one or more daily just to numb your senses from the pain you're feeling. If you drink for this reason, you will end up justifying it until you become an alcoholic before you can say lickety-split.

Take your medications being sure not to skip doses if you are on any. You can't be a good caregiver to your LO if your own health suffers.

Key # 9: Join a support group

You may not be able to picture yourself attending a support group but reconsider it. You will be surrounded by other family care-givers going through many of the same situations and experiencing emotions much like yours. They may have discovered ways of coping that never occurred to you.

Also, if your LO isn't bed-bound yet and is able to leave the house with help, you could develop a few friendships with people who would be willing to swap out a day with you now and then.

You could take your LO over to their house for them to watch in exchange for them coming over to yours.

Or, if your LO is bed-bound, you could make a similar arrangement with someone whose LO is still able to travel and you could sit for them in your home and then they could come to yours to help you out.

It's worth the effort. Stretch your borders and rediscover the outside world!

Key # 10: Pamper yourself

A minimum of once a week, treat yourself to a facial. Apply it just before you soak in a tub filled with hot, scented water, light some candles and put on soft instrumentals to play in the background.

Don't feel guilty pampering yourself while your LO is lying in the next room. You deserve a little time to yourself. Not only do you deserve it, you need it.

We have given you many suggestions in this chapter to help you plan a rewarding care-givers plan. Don't just read them. Implement them in this season of your life and when you have emerged from it, you will be the richer for it.

Chapter Ten
Open House:
A Joyful Farewell

I'd like to share my own mother's story with you to give you an alternative to a conventional funeral.

We've all heard it said before, and may have even said it ourselves, when someone dies, that they're in a better place or that they are out of pain now. These little colloquialisms have become the thing to say in an attempt to ease the pain of loss, however, when we are enlightened by the Lord about the reality of death and resurrection, there is very little or no grief at all. I know because I have experienced it personally. I have experienced His grace and mercy with the death of my own mother.

Please don't misunderstand me. I love my mother very, very much and I do miss her being here on Earth with me, but I am so happy for her and that joy overrides my own personal loss of her company. I eagerly anticipate my reunion with her.

As far as her spiritual background goes, she had a personal encounter with Jesus at an early age but remained private in her beliefs. I am the oldest child of four in the family and can't remember ever attending church with my parents growing up. They believed in God but we never discussed Him.

I accepted Jesus as my personal Lord and Savior twenty-five years ago and began witnessing to my family. Nine years later, mother asked me to pray for her to receive Jesus and then a year later, daddy asked me. Over the years, they prayed together on everything and Jesus became the focal point of their lives as they served Him with all their hearts.

Nine years ago, Mother was diagnosed with end stage lung disease due to a combination of smoking and undiagnosed walking pneumonia she had for three years. When she found out about the pneumonia, the damage to her lungs had already taken its toll. That was when she was first diagnosed with COPD and began having difficulty breathing. Over the years, she continued to stand in faith for her healing; always believing that the Lord loved her, had not abandoned her and was going to heal her. She never entertained the thought that God made her sick or that He refused to heal her. She was right. She is totally healed now.

Mother maintained her independence up until she had a stroke a few months ago and then she had to give up driving, but she still managed to shop for groceries and do little chores in their home with the help of Daddy and her portable oxygen. Then she started falling and bruising badly. Her healing process was slowed down because of the Coumadin she was prescribed after the stroke and years of steroids she had to take to help her breathe.

Finally, daddy realized he simply could not take care of her anymore at home and asked us to bring her to our home. This was such a difficult decision for him to make. After all, he had taken care of her for fifty-three years. I can honestly say that I never heard my parents raise their voices to each other or argue my entire life. They were each other's best friends and went everywhere and did everything together. When Daddy wasn't at work, he was home with us. He never drank, smoked or hung out with the boys and mother never went anywhere without Daddy, to speak of. They were so very in love and still are.

Just before coming to live with us, she had another bad fall and had to go to the hospital again. After being there three days, the pulmonologist told all of us that she only had thirty days to live. He said she could either check into their hospice unit or go home with me. She wanted me to take care of her. She said she trusted me implicitly and didn't want anyone else to care for her. I will always remember that she said that.

I was so happy to have her in my care at last so that I could lavish special love and attention on her and we made the most of our time together. After caring for dementia patients and the terminally ill in my own home for seventeen years and helping many families walk through the death, guilt and grief processes by ministering Jesus to them, it was the greatest honor of all to care for my own mother and be there for my family.

My daddy, Bob Turner, my husband, Bob, my sister, Debi Ursell, and my brother, Bob Turner Jr., spent time with her daily, talking about old times, feeding her and loving on her. The Lord gave us this precious time together as siblings, as well. We all appreciated each other and enjoyed pulling together for a common goal; to make mother's last days peaceful and joyful. Our sister, Janiece Hartmann, was unable to be with us as much because she lives in Dallas, but she visited when she could, which delighted our mother.

Vitas Hospice helped us with mothers' care in our home tremendously and she was assigned her own team which included an RN, social worker, chaplain, respiratory therapist, aide and their continuous care team. They displayed compassion coupled with experienced attentiveness to every detail of her needs and our family's concerns.

Two weeks before mother went on to be with the Lord, we held a living memorial (open house) for her in our home. Debi helped us plan it and made numerous calls, as did daddy, and sent as many emails out. It really paid off. One hundred and fifty friends and family members came to tell mother how she had changed their lives and what she meant to them and say goodbye. It was planned for two hours but went on for six hours. Mother took pictures with people, prayed, laughed and loved and then would nap between visitors. Many who attended hadn't seen mother and daddy for a long time. She was so loved and respected. It was glorious. There was such closure-such peace and total fulfillment. It was her last party and sendoff to heaven!

The day mother died and was resurrected, we flew our baby sister in from Dallas so that all of us would be with her at the end. I knew she was dying about noon that day and told daddy. He was very surprised because he thought she had improved over the last couple of weeks, but it was only an end of life rally. He spent some quality time alone with mother and then we all went into her room and sat around, laughing and talking about our childhood and occasionally, mother would smile at the stories, although her eyes were closed.

I had prepared her for death by telling her what was going to happen so that there would be no fear or panic at the end. We all prayed for her not to suffer and God was faithful to grant our petitions; she never did.

We were all there as she took her last peaceful breath at 1:30 a.m. and we praised our Creator as He welcomed her into her new, eternal home. We waved goodbye to her, knowing her soul left her body and floated up to the ceiling. I told her to be waiting for me in the light when my time came.

Then, we all prayed for one another and laid hands on daddy and prayed for him. There were some tears but not as you would expect when a beloved wife and mother dies so young (age 69). Immediately afterwards, the Lord moved me to cut locks of hair from her head and place them into individual zip lock bags and I kept one and distributed the rest to my siblings.

The funeral home came to pick her up and our family had sweet sleep that early morning, very satisfied that mother was literally in the Lords hands.

2 Co 5:8 "We are confident, yes, well pleased rather to be absent from the body and to be present with the Lord."

The next morning, we all came together at our home as a family and my sister, Debi, read several items mother had clipped from the newspaper and had instructed her to read the day following her death. Mother made prior arrangements to be cremated with no funeral following. The remains were to be returned to daddy.

A few days later, daddy came over to our home and gave me an old, yellowed envelope and some of my old baby pictures. The envelope also contained locks of the first haircut mother gave me as a baby.

Daddy always said that everything comes full circle; Mother gave me my first haircut and I gave mother her last. How amazing! I had both locks of hair framed and it hangs on our wall today as a memorial.

I realize that this is a very different way of handling death and a memorial service while the person is present and alive, with no funeral afterwards, but it was profoundly comforting. So much that Bob and I have decided this is the way we are going to handle our final arrangements if we have prior notice.

I also realized that Jesus had no funeral. He wasn't there. The women went to prepare His body according to their customs but He had risen.

"On the first day of the week, very early in the morning, the women took the spices they had prepared and went to the tomb. They found the stone rolled away from the tomb, but when they entered, they did not find the body of the Lord Jesus. While they were wondering about this, suddenly two men in clothes that gleamed like lightning stood beside them. In their fright the women bowed down with their faces to the ground, but the men said to them, "Why do you look for the living among the dead? He is not here; he has risen! Remember how he told you, while

he was still with you in Galilee: 'The Son of Man must be delivered into the hands of sinful men, be crucified and on the third day be raised again.'" Luke 24:1-7

The most amazing part of the end-of-life journey I took with my mother was that I never suffered any devastating grief when she left. I really believe that by celebrating her life while she was still here and making her a part of that celebration, it healed me. When it was all over, it was truly over. It helped, of course, that she was looking forward to being with the Lord. This gave all of us a great deal of peace; knowing she had no fear of death.

None of us missed having a traditional funeral and all that goes with it. We were actually relieved that there would be none. It would have worn us out emotionally and there was really no need for it after we had the living memorial with her.

What a marvelous inspiration my mother was to me. I now have total closure in every area, thanks to Jesus who saw me through every step of this journey.

Now, I'd like to share the details of our open house with you so if you want to do the same, you can build on our plan and customize your own.

Planning Your Open House

Get permission

First, talk to your dying LO about the idea to make sure he approves. Some people are extremely private and want to be left alone, so visitors aren't an option and you must respect and honor their wishes. If they agree with holding the living memorial/open house, gather together his spouse, your siblings and anyone else in his inner circle.

With your LO present, explain his wishes. Don't expect everyone to agree right away. It takes some getting used to; not having a funeral or graveside service after death. Most family members will want to adhere to your LO's requests but if someone in the crowd objects vehemently, give them time to digest it and, above all, don't fuss in front of your LO. Just drop it temporarily and then enlist the support of an agreeable family member to talk to him at another time away from your LO. When everyone is finally in agreement, proceed to the next step.

Plan the time & date

It will take time to go through your LO's address book and make your list and then send the invitations and emails and to make the follow-up calls so give yourself ample time to accomplish all of this. Don't try to do it all by yourself either; delegate!

You also must take into consideration how much time your LO has left and how ill he is. Ask his nurse or doctor how long they expect him to live. We planned two weeks in advance for mother's party and she passed away two weeks after the gathering so the timing was just right.

There will be those who can't make it on the date you finally decide on so tell them that instead, they can send him a letter or call him to express their gratitude for his being in their lives.

The time of day is also very important. We had ours after lunch so that the emphasis would be on mother instead of eating. We had chips, dip, cookies, horsedovers, tea and coffee set out. Make sure that you don't make the open house interfere with his care by scheduling it during a scheduled nursing visit or when the aide comes in to bathe him. His bath should be planned for that morning so he will be clean and fresh and all his linens are clean as well.

We held ours on a Saturday so the majority of people would be off work but you can plan yours whenever you feel that it would work for your LO, friends and family the best.

The Invitation

The wording of the invitation, whether you extend it verbally or in written form, should be done with great care so as not to hurt or offend others who may not agree with the idea of not holding a traditional funeral. For example:

You are invited to attend Virginia (Gin) Turner's Living Memorial Celebration! We have invited her friends and our family so all can express to her what she has meant to them during her lifetime and say their goodbyes for now. We encourage you to bring your camera to take a picture with her. The time is very short before she will go on to be with the Lord so she hopes to see you.

Day & Date: Saturday, August 19, 2006
Time: 2:00 p.m. – 5:00 p.m.
Location: 1234 Main Street
Hosted by: Starr & Bob Calo-oy
RSVP & directions: 521-8668

Though bed bound, Mother is in high spirits and her faith has kept her full of joy and eager anticipation, knowing she is heaven bound shortly!

Advance Preparations

There will be those who attend who cannot express their feelings verbally, especially in a crowded room, so:

1) Prepare a small, visible area close to the snacks with the following items:

- Small basket to contain folded notes
- Small tablet for writing a note to your LO
- A jar of pens
- A sign that reads "Feel free to write to (LO's name)"
- A guest book

2) Have your camera and camcorder charged and if you are too busy tending to the guests to do it yourself, delegate someone to take the pictures.

3) Have someone assigned in advance to answer the phone for you for last minute directions and someone else to answer the door.

4) Be sure to have plenty of Kleenex, chairs and toilet paper in place for the guests.

5) Have extra ice on hand.

6) If you have space, set up a room for those who need to grieve in private. Even though this is a celebration of your LO's life, grieving will be a natural thing to do for most of your guests so be sensitive to their needs.

Your job, as primary caregiver, is to make sure your LO does not get too tired or depressed and is not in pain. His comfort should be the most important thing to you. You are here for your LO-not the guests alone. Clear his room of visitors when you perform private care to preserve his dignity.

Karina's Story

I first met Karina Cardona, San Antonio Living television show producer in San Antonio, Texas, several years ago when she invited me to appear on the show to talk about my first book. Since then, we have stayed in touch so when I told her what we were going to do in regard to Mother's living memorial, she related to me the very special end of life celebration she and her family had for her dad this year. This is her story.

My Dad had been in the hospital since January 2006. Several times, in the months that followed, his doctors believed he was dying, so they told us to call family and friends to come pay their last respects. Each time he would miraculously come out of it, to everyone's surprise.

He was still in the hospital when we celebrated his 60th birthday (April 2006) after another close call. Two days before that, we didn't know if he would live to see another day, but he was blessed to celebrate another year of life. We wanted to make this birthday special, not just him, but for all of us who loved him.

All of the nurses knew that it was his birthday, so they wheeled his bed out of ICU and brought him out to the lobby. My entire family including my aunts, uncles, and grandfather were waiting with cake & pizza (even though he couldn't have any). We had a CD player with his favorite music, took pictures, and had everyone sign a frame for him. One of the nurses also took pictures and then gave us a poster board with my Dad's birthday pictures on it. It was a very special thing she did for us! We tacked it to the wall in his rehab room.

After his birthday, his condition improved significantly so they transferred him to rehab. He was doing so well that we were already talking about transferring him back home to Eagle Pass to finish out his rehab.

Just when we all thought that the worst had passed and he was going home, he was afflicted by a severe infection and never regained consciousness. We immediately called his brothers and sisters who live in Dallas and they made it down in a matter of hours, just in time to see him take his last breath. He passed, surrounded by those who had been with him since the beginning.

We took Dad home to Eagle Pass for his funeral so he made it back after all, just not the way we expected. Many people came over for the viewing all through the day and we ate and spent time together talking about old times. After the funeral – we had friends and family over again for the funeral reception and then most of them who were from out of town went back home.

I think for us, because there were so many close calls, we had several opportunities to say our 'goodbyes' to my Dad, so even though it happened suddenly, all of us were satisfied knowing we said most everything we needed to say. It was a gratifying ending for all of us who loved him.

We also took comfort in the fact that from January to May, there was never a day that he spent alone in the hospital. His wife, two daughters, son, grandkids, father, brothers, sisters, nieces, nephews, aunts, uncles, compadres and friends kept him company for the last five months of his life.

Our prayer for *you*, is that you plan a very special end-of-life celebration for your LO. Not that you have the same one we had for ours, but a very unique one for your entire family which will bring closure, peace and the satisfaction of knowing that it belonged to you and yours alone when all is said and done.

Chapter Eleven

Physical Signs of Impending Death

(Warning: this chapter is highly graphic but extremely necessary for the caregiver)

There are many times a dying person will simply pass away quietly in their sleep in the middle of the night. There may or may not have been warning that the time was near.

Other times, the entire family is there with them as they breathe their last breath.

We have taken care of terminally ill people in our home for many years and seen many deaths. We want to pass our experiences on to you now so you will be a little more prepared as to what happens before, during and after the death of your LO. You will, in turn, help your family members understand so that the dying process doesn't come as a shock to them.

When you notice a change in your LO, call his nurse immediately. Everyone has their own personal and unique way of leaving this world, but there are definite changes and some things all bodies go through when the shut-down process begins. Your LO may experience some, none or all of these changes. For example:

Drastic, Noticeable Changes

- He sleeps most of the time now.
- His breathing pattern radically changes.
- He is not aware of anyone in the room even though his eyes may be open. He doesn't respond to your touch or voice anymore.
- He can't/won't drink fluids anymore.
- He is not urinating or defecating like before.
- The urine output in his diaper or foley bag has mainly blood in it now.
- His room has a foul odor that is unidentifiable and you can't seem to locate or get rid of it.
- His feet and hands are getting cool/cold to the touch when they were usually warm before.
- He doesn't move anymore except while struggling to breathe.
- He has completely stopped talking or making any sounds.
- He stopped being combative and/or verbally abusive.
- He is talking to people in the room that you don't see.
- His skin color has changed.
- He doesn't want any visitors.
- He is extremely restless.

- He starts taking his clothes and/or diaper off and it isn't because he is hot.

His nurse will come over and take his vital signs and give you a report. In most cases, she will leave after the exam but if you want the hospice chaplain or social worker to come and wait with you, just tell her so she can arrange it. Call your pastor or priest and ask him to come over if he can, to support you and your family.

When the end is near you must realize that there is nothing anyone can do. All you can all do is wait for it to be over. There are no life-saving measures to be taken by hospice. They will make sure that your LO is comfortable and pain-free.

You also need to call anyone who asked to be there at the end.

Now is the time for you to say your last good-byes to your LO. This may be very hard for you to do, but you need to say it. Don't try to convince him to stay.

Hearing is the last sense to go, so even if he isn't able to respond to you by opening his eyes or squeezing your hand, still talk to him and tell him how much you love him. When everyone has said their good-byes and you are ready, tell your LO it's okay for him to depart. Sometimes that's all people need to let go.

Changes in communication

Your LO may be very sociable and talkative up until a few days before he dies but suddenly he stops talking- to anyone you can see anyway. He seems to be hallucinating and talking to people who aren't even there- or are they?

Throughout the centuries, there have been documented reports of dying people being visited by their dead relatives who had gone on before them. These conversations give us a glimpse into the world waiting for us when we go, so just listen, don't discourage or dismiss them.

Skin breakdown worsens

Your LO may have already been experiencing skin breakdown evidenced by bed sores on various parts of their body but toward the end, you will see more of it. It may seem that no matter how often you turn or reposition them, there is a new red or purple blotch every day now.

One reason for this is that the body is starting to shut down. The brain is not sending the skin repair commands to the skin and blood cells as it did before he got sick.

Also, your LO is not taking in liquids and food like he did before so now he is getting dehydrated and his skin does not have the hydration needed to remain healthy. All you can do at this point is to gently rub out any red spots and keep him turned every 2-3 hours around the clock. When he gets to the point that he cries or yells out in pain when you turn him or even touch him, stop turning him immediately.

Yes, that goes for baths too. I don't allow our patients' hospice home health aides to give them their baths anymore when they are nauseated, feverish or in pain. I keep their diaper area as clean as I can, taking care to move them as little as possible for even that. When they are this close, there is no reason to move them. There are, however, many reasons not to move them.

The skin may get worse when you stop turning him and he may develop a stronger odor just before the end, so light a strongly scented candle or incense or use a spray odor neutralizer in his room. Keep his bedclothes freshly changed and all garbage taken out immediately to cut down on odor and germs.

Another sign that the end is drawing near, is mottling. ***"Mottling" is a bluish or reddish marble-like pattern which appears on the skin, usually on the elbows, knees and feet.*** It moves up the feet to the ankles and the dying patient has usually expired by the time it reaches mid-thigh. This is caused by a lack of circulation when the blood begins to pool. The skin takes on a translucent appearance, feels very cold to the touch and mottling is very apparent. Not all people mottle though. It will be a combination of many signs when death is close.

Swallowing & choking problems develop

The body is truly amazing. Our spirit and soul are as well. They know when it is time to evacuate the body and so they begin the preparation for their departure from this earth.

The body says "I'm getting ready to shut down, so I will not permit any more food or liquid to enter me." When we try to "force" food or liquids at this point, the body chokes on the food because the esophagus stops working in compliance with the body's wishes. "Failure to thrive" is what the hospice calls this behavior.

If any liquid actually makes its way down, it goes into the wrong place. Instead of getting to the stomach, it goes into the lungs and then the body has to deal with pneumonia eventually which is accompanied by high fevers. This makes the dying so much more uncomfortable for the body.

When food or liquid gets shoveled in by a well meaning and loving caregiver, it will either go into the lungs or the stomach. If it goes into the lungs, the body will choke or vomit if there is still strength to do so. If not, the body may suffocate to death right then.

If it goes, and remains, in the stomach, the bowel has already shut down so the food just sits there and only gets partially digested. This is why the patient gets constipated and ceases from having bowel movements at the end. It won't do any good to administer laxative suppositories because the body won't react to them and all you will accomplish will be to make your LO more uncomfortable. It also won't help to give suppositories for fever for the same reason.

The reason that some dying people swell up in their extremities, such as their hands and feet, is because the body is holding on to any liquid left because it "knows" there won't be any more permitted to come into it and it uses what's there to keep cooling itself as much as possible, to the very end.

This is one reason that the urine output decreases, usually turns dark red with old blood and then stops altogether.

Breathing problems become more apparent

The body is starting to shut down all of its organs so the lungs have to work harder to get oxygen to all of the existing blood cells. This causes a dramatic increase in respirations. Another reason for the increase is that if the patient has pneumonia and/or the lungs start to fill up.

"Respiration" is the term used for each breath taken. The normal number of respirations per minute is 16-18. This number usually increases in the dying person to as high as 60 per minute! We have seen some of our patients go on like this, day and night, for as long as three days until their heart finally gave out.

The Death Rattle

When death is coming very soon, the death rattle begins. This sound is a result of mucous trapped in the throat. Hospice will provide Atropine drops to place under your LO's tongue to silence the gurgling by helping to dry it up.

When the end is only a few hours away, the dying patient will start pausing between breaths. Respirations go down to between 6-8 per minute, then 4-5, and then finally stop completely. In many cases we have seen the family grieving the death of their loved one for 1-2 minutes when all of a sudden, their LO breathes one last time. This can be startling to the family, to say the least.

These are the most common signs of impending death.

The most important things to remember is not to panic, comfort your LO and enjoy the last few days or hours he is with you as best you can.

The Don'ts

- Don't try to get him to talk when he doesn't want to.
- Don't correct him when he says something that isn't true.
- Don't try to force him to eat or drink by manipulating or threatening him.
- Don't force him to stay awake when he wants to sleep.
- Don't force medication on him if he can't swallow it.
- Don't try to force family members to sit with him or to even go into his room if they don't want to.
- Don't ask him questions about anything.
- Don't sob loudly in his presence.
- Don't talk about funeral plans with others in his presence.
- Don't argue with others in his presence.
- Don't withhold his pain medication because you are worried that he'll get addicted.

- Don't suffer through this alone. Hospice is there to help you. Just ask.

<u>The Do's:</u>

- Do swab his mouth twice per hour with mouth swabs.
- Do stroke his hair gently.
- Do kiss him and tell him you love him and that you are there for him.
- Do keep an eye out for any part of his body that touches something hard to avoid bedsores.
- Do keep his bedding and clothing dry especially if he's perspiring.
- Do get your rest.
- Do eat and stay well hydrated yourself.
- Do take breaks and allow others to stay with him so you can get out of the room or the house.

We aren't just filling page space with all of these suggestions. Please read and re-read these points and then take them to heart and apply them. They can definitely make the difference from you getting burned out emotionally and physically and/or you're helping your LO make this final passage of his life easier.

Chapter Twelve

The Day My Loved One Dies

It's hard to wrap your mind around the fact that after all of the work, the waiting, the struggling, the ups and downs, mixed emotions, anger, regret, resolutions, feelings of resentment toward those who weren't there to help out and then the forgiveness and the resignation, that he is really gone.

Humans work for reward at the end of a job well done and we can physically see the results which makes our hearts swell up with pride. What do you do with you're your emotions when the end result of caring for your loved one is death? Death = failure in most peoples minds, but not in this case. You have unquestionably succeeded in your mission of mercy and love.

But you ask yourself, "How can I stand back from his bed now and receive my pats on the back? Where is the applause?" This is one of the main reasons it's so hard to go through the death of a loved one when you have been the primary caregiver. After the funeral home takes away the very object of your sacrifice and tedious, vigilant work all of this time, you are left at home with an empty bed.

Let me put all of this into proper perspective for you. No, you don't have a newly tiled floor to stand back and admire. Instead, you take away with you great satisfaction that you were there all the way through the wound dressings, diaper changes, baths, hand holding, head stroking and that you did it exquisitely as if it were you lying in that bed. God saw and appreciates what you did, even if no one else on earth does and His admiration is really all that counts.

It is totally natural for you to feel a sense of relief so don't add to that the toxic element of guilt. True, there will be a void in your life for a while because for this season in your life, your every waking hour has been spent focusing on life and death issues and now it's suddenly over. What are you going to do with your time now?

You may have dreamed of all of the things you'd rather be doing than caring for him, but now that he is gone, you'd give anything for one more diaper to change. This is normal to feel this way but cut yourself some slack- no one can be "on" all the time and you did the very best you could. Appease yourself with the fact that you finished the race and then be proud of yourself. Many people cannot do what you did or even attempt it. Congratulations!

After the initial shock has passed and you catch your breath, there are still some details that must be taken care of. Gather up all of his medications and put them in a zip-lock bag to hand over to the hospice nurse when she asks for them a little later.

What Will Happen

Your LO has just died and there are family members, including yourself, standing and sitting all around the house crying and holding each other. Now what do you do? The answer is anything you want to do. It's finally over. It may take some time to really sink in, but it is over now.

Do not move your LO's body in any way. Do not turn the oxygen concentrator off. The nurse will do this when she pronounces him dead and records the time. Do not change his clothing, diaper or sheets. Leave everything as is for now. In a little while, the nurse will call the police (this is routine) and they will come over to investigate and eliminate foul play.

Sometimes, a police detective comes also and he will ask everyone to wait in the living room while he goes into your LO's room, closes the door and makes his report.

If the nurse isn't there when he passes away, call hospice and they will page her to come over. She will make all the necessary calls when she gets there.

You should make any calls you want to on another line but leave your main line clear for the barrage of calls that will be coming in and going out over the next few hours by the medical personnel in your home. If you receive a personal call, tell the caller to call you on another line such as a cell phone or fax line if possible. If you don't have another phone available, talk to them very briefly and tell them you'll call them back after everyone leaves.

What the Nurse Will Do When She Arrives

- Call the doctor who is to sign the death certificate. This could be either his personal doctor or the hospice doctor.

- Call the medical examiner to let him know who will be signing the death certificate.

- Call the police and report the death.

- Call the funeral home after the police leave.

- Check the medications and have you witness and sign off to her emptying the narcotics into the toilet.

- Call the medical equipment supplier to have them come out to pick up the hospital bed, oxygen concentrator or any other equipment they brought out for your LO.

- Sit down and fill out her report.

- Give a verbal report to the police.

After she is finished with her responsibilities, she will stay with you until the funeral home gets there to pick up your LO if you want her to. If you don't need her, tell her that she can leave so she can make the rest of her visits for the day.

Before the funeral home gets there, get his dentures ready (make sure they are clean) his glasses, any framed pictures you want put out the day of the funeral and lay out his funeral clothes for them to take along with him.

Death Certificates

Make sure that you order at least six copies of his death certificate. They will be required for:

1. banks
2. pensions
3. The Veterans Administration
4. Life insurance companies
5. His credit card agencies
6. Extras, just in case

Whenever you want for your family and friends to leave, just tell them you need to do the paperwork and that you will let them know what time to be at the funeral home- that you are going to go over there as soon as you're finished and make the final arrangements. You may want someone else to go in your stead if you are too exhausted. If so, don't hesitate to ask. You are going to have to tell them that it is over-they can leave-there is nothing else for them to do. Maybe they want to all get together and go eat if they have been putting off eating until it was over. If you want someone to stay with you, ask them.

What You Are To Do

What you do after the funeral home leaves with your LO is up to you. You don't have to go to the funeral home right away if you don't want to. You may just want to rest first or take a long, hot bath or shower and then sleep for a while. You may be restless and just want to clean his room. You may want to just be alone. Do what you want to do- period! You have done the very best you could do as the primary caregiver and now your LO has gone on to be with Jesus. You will be rewarded greatly for all of your hard work and close attention to the many details that came with being a caring caregiver. Get your rest because you are going to have a few more days of paperwork and tough decisions to make regarding your LO's estate and funeral preparations and you'll need your strength.

Chapter Thirteen
What to do When You Come Home from the Funeral

The caregiving, funeral and reception is over now and you are alone with your memories of your LO. Now, what do you do?

You aren't the same person you were before all of this first began. You are wiser, more patient and compassionate, and hopefully, have mercy for all who are in the world now.

You need to recuperate for a while without any demands being made on your time by anyone. If you have your own family, they are bound to be happy to have you to themselves again.

After you have gotten some rest and are ready to tackle it, it's time to gather up all of your LO's things and decide what to do with them. If he left behind any valuables at your home, his will should designate who gets what.

Make sure the medical equipment supplier comes to pick up their things.

What did you do before the caregiving? Did you have a job outside of your home? Do you want it back? If so, pursue it.

Were you more involved in your children's lives? Then visit with them to see what they are doing these days and would they like some company or help.

Of course, you don't really have to DO anything but there will be a void caused by your LO's death that may feel a little uncomfortable for a while.

To grieve for a while is completely normal. To miss your LO forever is also, but to grieve uncontrollably but for it to take over your life and interfere with your ability to concentrate on anything is not normal.

Make a list (yes, just one more!) of your goals and your interests. Write down any obstacles that could possibly arrive to prevent you from achieving them. Write down a plan to attaining them and then a date to begin pursuing them and then go after them!

You have done a marvelous job with your LO and should be very proud of yourself! Some day, when you need a compassionate caregiver, God will see to it that you are compensated for all the good caregiving seed you have sown and you will reap bountifully.

We hope that the information in our book has helped you to be a caring caregiver!

Sources & Resources for the Family Caregiver

The Caring Caregiver (for advice re: caregiving)
210-521-8668
www.caregiversadvice.net **(our website)**

The Guide to Good Care by Gilberto Garza Jr.
www.theguidetogoodcare.com

Alzheimer's Association
800-272-3900
www.alz.org

Advice & comfort to family caregivers
www.geocities.com/pandora2000/Caregiving.html

BoomerBooks.com (practical knowledge and solutions for dealing with family, retirement and aging that arrive after age 50 whether you're ready or not.
www.boomer-books.com

Caregiver.com (today's online caregiver magazine)
www.caregiver.com

The Caregivers Companion (joining your fellow caregivers in a very challenging and important journey)
www.caregivercompanion.com

Caregiving.com (solutions to your caregiving situations throughout the caregiving years)
www.caregiving.com

Caregiving tips for family caregivers – non-commercial, consumer friendly expert information on mental health and aging.
www.helpguide.org

The Careguide (Everything families need to understand, plan and manage care for their elderly loved one.
www.careguide.com

Children of Aging Parents – a non-profit, charitable organization whose mission is to assist the nation's nearly 54 million caregivers of the elderly and chronically ill with reliable information, referrals and support; to heighten public awareness that the health of the family caregiver is essential to ensure quality care of the nation's growing elderly population.
www.caps4caregivers.org

www.elderrage.com – A *terrific* website by Jacqueline Marcell; Eldercare / Alzheimer's Speaker, Author, Radio Host, Caregiver Advocate

Eldercare Online – A beacon for people caring for aging loved ones.
www.ec-online.net

Empowering Caregivers – Provides an opportunity to look at many of the issues that caregivers may be experiencing.
www.care-givers.com

Geriatric Resources – A company specializing in caregiving resources and services for those suffering from Alzheimer's disease.
www.geriatric-resources.com

Hospice foundation of America – Contains links to frequently requested information about hospice.
www.hospicefoundation.org

National Association for Home Care – Committed to representing the interests of the home care and hospice community.
www.nahc.org

National Hospice Foundation – Contains links to better your understanding about hospice and palliative care.
www.nhpco.org

The Ribbon Online- A website inspired by The Ribbon Newsletter, created to provide information to caregivers dealing with Alzheimer's disease and dementia.
www.theribbon.com

Top Alzheimer's/Caregiving Sites – 150 top Alzheimer websites in order of their ranking

position. Loaded with message boards, tips & advice on all types of caregiving, memorials etc. http:/new.topsitelists.com/bestsites/bpsibley/topsites.html

Foundation for Hospice & Home Care

202-547-6586

Works to improve public policy on health care, particularly for the elderly. They help the family to select a good hospice agency and provide them with referrals to local organizations that offer home care.

Hospice Association of America

202-546-4759

The family caregiver is provided with videos, brochures and books on hospice care and this organization makes referrals to local agencies.

www.hospice-america.org

Hospice Helpline

National Hospice Organization

800-658-8898

Glossary

A

- **actively dying** – An individualized process of dying.
- **agitation** – When a person becomes overly excited or disturbed.
- **alcohol related dementia** – Dementia brought about by the excessive use of alcohol.
- **Alzheimer's Disease** – A progressive, irreversible disease characterized by degeneration of the brain cells and leading to severe dementia.
- **ambulatory** – The ability to walk and move around.
- **aspirating** – To suck or inhale fluid into the lungs.
- **atropine** – A drug used shortly before death, to dry up the terminal secretions in the throat which make the "death rattle" sounds.

B

- **bed-bound** – When a person can no longer get up from their bed due to health problems.
- **bereavement** – the period after a loss during which grief is experienced and mourning occurs. The time spent in a period of bereavement depends on how

attached the person was to the person who died, and how much time was spent anticipating the loss.

- **burn-out** – A state of emotional exhaustion caused by an overload of care-giving, work and other responsibilities.

C

- **catastrophic reaction** – When a dementia victim has been over stimulated, angered, startled or frightened, many times their reaction will be to scream, spit, kick, yell, pinch, strike out at others or exhibit other inappropriate behavior.
- **cognition** – the area of more sophisticated mental functioning (intelligence, judgment, insight, memory and so on).
- **combativeness** – When the dementia victim strikes back physically at anyone within reach.
- **confusion** – Failure to distinguish between things. A state of disorder.
- **congestive heart failure** – Weakness of the heart muscle that leads to a buildup of fluid in body tissues (such as legs, lungs, liver). The condition is caused when the heart is unable to pump enough blood to meet the needs of the body.
- **cremation** – the burning of a dead body until only ashes are left.

D

- **death certificate** – a document proclaiming the death of an individual and cause of death.
- **dehydration** – When a person has lost too much water in their body and they have become dry.
- **delusions** – A belief in something that is contrary to fact or reality as a result of dementia.
- **dementia** – partial or total loss of personality and other significant mental functions such as memory capacity, severe enough to interfere with social or occupational functioning, but without psychosis.
- **depilatory cream** – A substance that removes unwanted hair.
- **depression** – an unpleasant, unhappy state of mind and body with significant impairment of memory, concentration and other mental processes. Physical activity is also slowed.
- **diagnosis** – the identifying of an illness or disorder through an interview, physical examination, and medical tests and other treatments.
- **disoriented** – feeling lost or confused, especially with regard to direction or position.

- **DNR** – "Do not resuscitate." Not using any artificial means to keep someone alive. Comfort and palliative care only.
- **durable power of attorney for health care** – document allowing others to make health care decisions when one is not able to. Also called health care power of attorney or health care directive.

E

- **eulogy** – a speech or piece of writing that praises somebody or something very highly, especially a tribute to somebody who has recently died.
- **executor** – is the person or institution named in a person's will who carries out the terms of the will. Traditionally, the word has referred to the male and Executrix to the female, but this distinction is rapidly disappearing.

F

- **financial planning** – planning relating to or involving money or finance.
- **funeral reception** – a gathering, consisting of family and friends, held at a particular location after a funeral.

G

- **grief** – from the same root as grave, aggravate, baritone. Mental anguish, annoyance, regret, trouble, grievance.
- **grief counselor** – an educated person in the area of grief that helps people through their pain following a death.
- **grief therapist** – a licensed therapist who specializes in the grief process.

H

- **hallucination - Seeing** something that is not there.
- **home health** – When a patient meets the medical requirements necessary to receive nursing care in their home, funded through Medicare, a home health agency is assigned by the patient's doctor. A registered nurse comes to the patient's home or a personal care home, usually weekly, to take their vital signs and check their body. Home health also provides, with the doctor's approval, a home health aide who gives the patient a bath, mouth care, changes bed clothes for them and cleans their nails, shaves them and shampoos their hair. The agency also provides services by making

available to the patient, a chaplain, social worker, therapy and case management. The length and frequency of the visits from each department vary according to their needs, but none of these people stay with the patient in their home.

- **hospice** – There are times when the family of a terminally ill person no longer has the ability or energy to care for them at home but they don't want them to spend their final days in a hospital, nursing home or any other medical facility. A hospice is a home away from home for the sick and/or dying and provides the perfect alternative. Some personal care homes specialize in hospice patients.
- **hospice agency** – A home health agency whose sole purpose is to provide support to the family and patient and care for the terminally ill; physically, mentally, spiritually and emotionally.
- **hydration** – to provide water for something or somebody in order to reestablish or maintain a correct fluid balance.

I

- **incontinence** – When a person becomes unable to restrain a natural discharge, such as urine or feces, from leaving their body.
- **inflammation** – the body's reaction to injury. Signs of inflammation are redness, heat, swelling and tenderness.
- **interdisciplinary team** – A group of individuals with varying areas of specialty assembled to solve a problem or perform a task. The team is assembled out of recognition that no one discipline is sufficiently broad enough to adequately analyze the problem and propose action.

L

- **living trust** – is a trust set up to operate during the life (and can operate after the death) of the one setting up the trust. It can be revocable, or, in other words, you can change your mind and have some or all of the trust property returned to you during your life. An irrevocable trust cannot be changed except in certain legal circumstances (fraud, unlawful agreements, merger of interests, and decision of the Court).

- **living will** – a will that asks to not be kept alive by life support.
- **lucid** – rational and mentally clear, especially only for a period between episodes of delirium or psychosis.

M

- **malnutrition** – the lack of healthy foods in the diet or an excessive intake of unhealthy foods, leading to physical harm.
- **memorial service** – like a funeral, except not in the presence of the body.
- **moisture barrier ointment** – a petroleum based protectant for the skin which keeps moisture from coming in contact with the skin.
- **mottling** – When the blood pools in the extremities of the body just prior to death.

N

- **nebulizer** – a device used to give drugs through a powered air pump which converts a liquid to a fine spray for inhalation.
- **non-ambulatory**- Not being able to walk or move around.

- **nursing home**-A facility equipped and staffed to provide care for the infirm, chronically ill and disabled.

P

- **palliative care** – Care given to improve the quality of life of patients who have a serious or life-threatening disease. The goal of palliative care is to prevent or treat as early as possible the symptoms of the disease, side effects caused by treatment of the disease, and psychological, social, and spiritual problems related to the disease or its treatment. Also called comfort care, supportive care, and symptom management.
- **pallbearers** – somebody who helps to carry or escort a casket at a funeral or burial.
- **paranoia** – a psychiatric disorder involving systemized delusion, usually of persecution.
- **pathologist** – study of disease, the manifestation of disease, departure from normality.
- **power of attorney**-A written statement legally authorizing a person to act for another.
- **pneumonia** – an inflammation of one or both lungs, usually caused by infection from a

bacterium or virus or, less commonly, by a chemical or physical irritant.

- **private or personal care home**-A residential care home that cares for the elderly or terminally ill, as an alternative to placement in a nursing home.
- **probate** – is the legal process of proving a will, appointing an executor, and settling an estate; but by custom, it has come to be understood as the legal process whereby a dead person's estate is administered and distributed.

S

- **sitter**-A person hired to supervise and take care of someone.
- s**ocial skills**-Having the ability to behave mannerly or politely in public without fear or incident.
- **social worker**-A counselor that specializes in promoting the welfare of the dementia victim and their family by way of providing information.
- **support group**-A group of people who share a similar set of problems or circumstances that meet at a designated time and place to share and give support to one another.

T

- **thickeners**- A powder such as "Thickett" that when mixed with a liquid, becomes thick enough for the person with swallowing difficulties to be able to drink better, hopefully without choking.
- **trust** – is defined as any arrangement where property is to be held and administered by a trustee for the benefit of those for whom the trust was created. Depending on the type and how it is established, a trust may be revocable (changeable) or irrevocable (not changeable).
- **turning**-When the terminally ill, bed bound patient must be turned from side to side at particular time intervals to avoid getting bedsores.

W

- **will** – is the legal expression or declaration of a person's mind or wishes as to the disposition of the person's property, to be performed or take effect after the person's death.

- **word finding problems**-When the dementia victim uses incorrect words to express their thoughts, feelings or desires.

About the Authors
Starr & Bob Calo-oy,

"Hospice Care at Home"

Bob & Starr Calo-oy were both born and raised in San Antonio and have been married for 26 years.

For the past 17 years, they have owned and operated a personal care home specializing in the care of terminally ill patients and victims of Alzheimer's disease and other forms of dementia in their San Antonio home.

In addition to caring for the elderly in their home, they give in-service training for doctors, nurses, the staffs of hospices and home health agencies, sharing tips and unique ideas for caring for dementia victims. Starr also gives private consultations to individuals on how to start and operate a successful personal care home.

Starr is past Vice-President of San Antonio Residential Care Homes (SARCH) and was the creator, editor and publisher of their newsletter from 1998 through 2001. She is also past Vice President, editor and publications director on the board of *The Final Draft,* the newsletter for the San Antonio Writers Guild.

Starr is a columnist for SAWorship.com as well as a free lance writer for the San Antonio Express-News.

In April 2004, they released their first book, "*The Caring Caregivers Guide to Dealing with Guilt",* about the experiences they've had over 17 years of operating their personal care home. This book is about the undeserved guilt families experience when they turn the care of their loved ones over to someone else. However, if the family desires to care for their loved one in their own home, it provides tips and directions to help them. It is written so that the medical field can benefit by empathizing while at the same time making it easy for the non-medical professional to easily understand its content.

They published their own monthly, 20-page tabloid newspaper, the ***TELESTARR***, which was circulated throughout South Texas city, county and state agencies for eight years.

They also counsel couples to help them to develop a more meaningful relationship and better communication skills.

They have also written a series of booklets to help the family caregiver, having to do with the different dilemmas that the family caregiver faces when caring for their loved one. (these can be purchased in the back pages of this book)

Starr and Bob speak at conventions, seminars, civic clubs, health care facilities, and make television and radio appearances.

Recommended Reading

1) **36-Hour Day**: A Family Guide to Caring for Persons with Alzheimer Disease, Related Dementing Illnesses, and Memory Loss in Later Life
Nancy L. Mace, Peter V. Rabins

2) **Sacred Passage**: How to Provide Fearless, Compassionate Care for the Dying
Margaret Coberly Ph.D, RN

3) **A Good Death**: Challenges, Choices, and Care Options by Charles Meyer

4) **Handbook for Mortals**: Guidance for People Facing Serious Illness
Joanne Lynn, Joan Harrold

5) **Caring for Patients at the End of Life**: Facing an Uncertain Future Together
Timothy E. Quill

6) **Family Handbook of Hospice Care**
Fairview Health Services

7) **How to Care for Aging Parents**
Virginia Morris, Foreword by Robert M. Butler

8) **Complete Eldercare Planner**: Where to Start, Which Questions to Ask, and how to Find Help
Joy Loverde

9) **Home Care for the Elderly**: An International Perspective
Abraham Monk, Carole Cox

10) **Don't Put Me in a Nursing Home**: Dr Amarnick Responds to Every Elder's Silent Plea
Claude Amarnick

11) **Home Care Companion's Quick Tips for Caregivers**
Marion Karpinski R.N., Don Thomas (Illustrator)

12) **Eldercare for Dummies**
Rachelle Zukerman

13) **And Thou Shalt Honor**: The Caregiver's Companion
Beth Witrogen McLeod (Editor), Bob Condor

14) **Healing a Spouse's Grieving Heart**: 100 Practical Ideas After Your Husband or Wife Dies: Compassionate Advice and Simple Activities for Windows and Widowers
Alan D. Wolfelt

15) **When Someone You Love Is Dying**
David Clark, Peter Emmett

16) **Dying at Home**: A Family Guide for Caregiving
Andrea Sankar

17) **Helping Yourself Help Others**: A Book for Caregivers
Rosalynn Carter, Susan K. Golant

18) **American Medical Association Guide to Home Caregiving**
American Medical Association, Angela Perry (Editor)

A

B

C

D

E

F

G

H

I

L

M

N

P

S

T

W

"The Caring Caregivers Guide to Dealing with Guilt" by Starr & Bob Calo-oy

Do you suffer with one or more of these types of guilt?

- **Guilt resulting from a broken promise**
- **Guilt resulting from physical abuse**
- **Guilt as a result of sibling abuse**
- **Guilt resulting from revengeful thoughts and unforgiveness**
- **Guilt resulting from wanting your loved one to die**
- **Guilt resulting from a hardened heart**
- **Guilt resulting from emotionally not being able to visit**
- **Guilt resulting from mixed emotions**

If so, you will find solutions in this truly remarkable guide to caregiver guilt.

Also included…

- **Unique and creative caregiving tips**
- **The Stages the family goes through**
- **FAQ section**
- **Suggestions at the end of each chapter for dealing with specific guilt**

Whether you are a family caregiver, a physician, nurse, social worker, case manager or with the clergy, you will benefit greatly with the rich advice and practical applications in this marvelous guide.

Easy Order Form

Please send ____copies of the Orchard Publication:

"Hospice Care at Home"

Please send ____copies of the Orchard Publication:

"The Caring Caregivers Guide to Dealing with Guilt"

Each book costs $21.36 which includes tax (plus shipping). SHIPPING: *US:* Add $4.00 for the first book and $2.00 for each additional book.

Other Publications by Starr Calo-oy

The following booklets (small books) are highly informative and easy to read because of their size. They make great gifts too! Collect them all! All booklets cost only $7.00 each including tax, S&H.

1. Ten Keys to Avoiding Caregiver Burnout
2. Creative Tips When Dealing with Angry & Paranoid People with Dementia
3. Family Caregiving Tips, Hands-On
4. The Tip Book- Medical Problems of the Bed Bound Person
5. Elderly Behavioral Problems- Volume 1
6. Elderly Behavioral Problems- Volume 2
7. How to Plan a Funeral for Your Loved One

Hospice Care at Home

Please send the following booklets (ex. 1,2,3, etc.)

____

PHONE: (210) 521-8668 ***(Have your credit card ready)***

FAX: (210) 979-0900

WEBSITE: www.caregiversadvice.net

Name:______________________________

E-mail:______________________________

Address:____________________________

City:_______________________________

St.____Zip__________________________

Phone: (___)_________________________

Name on card:_______________________

Account Number:_____________________

Expiration Date:______________________

Three digit number on back of card:______

Signature:___________________________

Or mail check or money order to:
Orchard Publications
P.O. Box 680815
San Antonio, Texas 78268

MBK Homecare Consultations

Start your own care home!

So, you want to start your own residential homecare business for the elderly but you really don't know where to start or how to do it. Within hours I can have you fully equipped to walk out of my home with a referral base, get your first client and start making money regardless of your education. You do not have to hold any specific degrees. All you really need is a love for the elderly, a servant's heart, patience and a desire to provide an excellent alternative to nursing home care. In short, you become an extension your client's family.

Adult children and spouses become caregivers every day in their own homes and so can you. I have done homecare consultations for the past 16 years and helped numerous people become homecare providers.

If you will fill out the MBK questionnaire on-line prior to my calling you for an appointment, I can custom design your interview to fit your particular personality, background, capabilities and desires.

I have listed below the topics on which I will educate you and instruments that I will provide you with during the interview:

- The phone interview with the family- how to screen them for: their ability to pay, the type of client as to make a perfect match re: caregiver to resident, their ability to conform to your house rules, any future problems that could develop re: family dynamics.
- How to decide what type of client you have the ability and desire to take on. You may want to specialize in dementia victims or the terminally ill, head injury patients or the mentally

challenged, brain tumor, cancer, paraplegic, quadriplegic, ambulatory and well-minded or other not mentioned here.

- How to set up your home to care for specific patients.
- Menus, meal plans, special diets, tips on how to feed someone, swallowing problems and how to deal with them.
- How to help the family of an elderly loved one convince them to leave their home and move in with you.
- How to get the best prices on medical supplies.
- How to prepare your monthly billing statements and what to charge for.
- Activities for your residents.
- Referral sources
- The rules regarding an unlicensed facility
- Various forms
- Dealing with nursing agencies
- Social workers
- How to screen your hired help and what you need for your type facility
- The difference between private/semi-private
- Injections, medications and special medical equipment
- Supplies and grocery shopping
- Outings, going home for the day
- Special diets, liquid supplements, Thickett
- Pets, color therapy, aromatherapy, water therapy
- Supply deposits and monthly fees
- Special services: Hair done in the home, podiatrists, lab work, nail care, facials, rubdowns
- Monthly family reports

Hospice Care at Home

- Your floor plan-how to make it work for you
- The different types of families you will encounter
- Preventing negative family dynamics
- Visiting hours and days
- Dealing with the doctors and nurses
- Preparing your bathrooms
- Safety measures
- Keeping the air clean smelling in your home
- Monthly family parties
- Pre-visit doctor reports
- Setting up the client's folder
- In the event of death
- Holidays and other special occasions
- Dealing with denial
- How to make it their home

I charge only $100.00 per hour to give you everything listed above and depending on our conversation apart from the teaching.

Make an investment in your future! If this sounds like something you might be interested in doing with your life, call me today so I can help you get on your way to a very rewarding career.

Starr Calo-oy

210-521-8668

www.caregiversadvice.net